Scientific research involving human embryos was a major topic of public debate in Britain during the 1980s. Despite strong support from the scientific community, embryo research was initially condemned by many ordinary people as well as by special interest groups, and came close to being banned by Act of Parliament. Michael Mulkay describes the dynamics of the parliamentary struggle over the future of embryo research, focusing on such issues as: the clash between the anti-abortion and pro-research lobbies; the tactics of the Government; political ideology; the media's role; the importance of gender; religion; the impact of science fiction; the lure of medical advance; and the difficulty of maintaining ethical control. He explains how the advocates of embryo research eventually triumphed, and ends with an examination of the cultural tensions that linger after the debate.

The embryo research debate

Cambridge Cultural Social Studies

General editors: JEFFREY C. ALEXANDER, *Department of Sociology, University of California, Los Angeles, and* STEVEN SEIDMAN, *Department of Sociology, University at Albany, State University of New York.*

Editorial Board
JEAN COMAROFF, *Department of Anthropology, University of Chicago*
DONNA HARAWAY, *Department of the History of Consciousness, University of California, Santa Cruz*
MICHELE LAMONT, *Department of Sociology, Princeton University*
THOMAS LAQUEUR, *Department of History, University of California, Berkeley*

Titles in the series
ILANA FRIEDRICH SILBER, *Virtuosity, charisma, and social order*
LINDA NICHOLSON AND STEVEN SEIDMAN (eds.), *Social postmodernism*
WILLIAM BOGARD, *The simulation of surveillance*
SUZANNE R. KIRSCHNER, *The religious and Romantic origins of psychoanalysis*
PAUL LITCHTERMAN, *The search for political community*
ROGER FRIEDLAND AND RICHARD HECHT, *To rule Jerusalem*
KENNETH H. TUCKER, *French revolutionary syndicalism and the public sphere*
ERIK RINGMAR, *Identity, interest and action*
ALBERTO MELUCCI, *The playing self*
ALBERTO MELUCCI, *Challenging codes*
SARAH M. CORSE, *Nationalism and literature*
DARNELL M. HUNT, *Screening the LA riots*
LYNETTE P. SPILLMAN, *Nation and commemoration*

The embryo research debate

Science and the politics of reproduction

Michael Mulkay
University of York

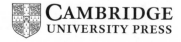

CAMBRIDGE
UNIVERSITY PRESS

Published by the Press Syndicate of the University of Cambridge
The Pitt Building, Trumpington Street, Cambridge CB2 1RP
40 West 20th Street, New York, NY 10011–4211, USA
10 Stamford Road, Melbourne 3166, Australia

First published 1997

Printed in Great Britain at the University Press, Cambridge

A catalogue record for this book is available from the British Library

Library of Congress cataloguing in publication data

Mulkay, M. J. (Michael Joseph), 1936–
    The embryo research debate : science and the politics of
reproduction / Michael Mulkay.
        p.   cm. – (Cambridge cultural social studies)
    Includes bibliographical references and index.
    ISBN 0-521-57180-4 (hc). – ISBN 0-521-57683-0 (pb)
    1. Human reproductive technology – Political aspects – Great
Britain.   2. Human embryo – Research – Political aspects – Great
Britain.   I. Title.   II. Series.
RG133.5.M846   1997
176'.0941–dc20   96–29109   CIP

ISBN 0 521 57180 4 hardback
ISBN 0 521 57683 0 paperback

For Lucy

Contents

Preface and acknowledgements

The main text of this book takes the form of a historical narrative, based upon close examination of documentary records, which tells the story of the public debate over embryo research in Britain. I have tried to provide a richly descriptive account of the debate which is informed by the relevant academic literature, but which is not encumbered by constant reference to academic issues and which is directly accessible to readers with no knowledge of that literature.

A straightforward narrative form is well suited to the topic of the embryo research debate. But it is by no means the only formal framework that may be used to throw light on this sequence of events. Indeed, my first, preliminary, attempt to explore the debate was written in the quite different form of a dream fantasy. I have included this alternative portrayal as an epilogue to the main text, in the hope that its unusual format will encourage readers to examine their own views on the social and moral significance of scientific research involving human embryos, and to reflect on the story presented in the preceding chapters.

This book re-examines, and places in a wider context, some of the findings I have presented in a series of articles published between 1993 and 1996. Several of the topics covered in those articles have been omitted from the book, however, whilst some of the arguments have been revised and a substantial amount of new material has been introduced. In other words, the series of articles and the book differ considerably in scope and in content.

I wish to thank the following people for their encouragement and for helping me in various concrete ways: Kenneth Boyd, Daniel Callahan, David Edge, Alan Handyside, Henry Leese, Lucy Mulkay, Jack Scarisbrick and Steven Yearley. I also thank the Economic and Social Research Council for awarding me a grant for the years 1992–4 (R 000 23 3722), during which time I carried out most of the detailed research on the embryo research debate; and the Warden and Fellows of Nuffield College, Oxford, who elected me to a Norman Chester Senior Research Fellowship for the Michaelmas term 1995, and thereby enabled me to bring the work to completion. In addition, I am grateful to the anonymous referee who examined the complete manuscript of this study with great care and whose comments were most helpful.

I thank Professor R. G. Edwards, the editor of *Human Reproduction*, for granting me permission to reproduce 'Intruders in the fallopian tube or a dream of perfect human reproduction', which was first published in *Human Reproduction* 6 (1991), 1480–6. I thank IOP Publishing Ltd and the editor of *Public Understanding of Science* for allowing me to draw upon the following of my articles: 'Embryos in the news', 3 (1994), 33–51; 'Changing minds about embryo research', 3 (1994), 195–213; 'Political parties, parliamentary lobbies and embryo research', 4 (1995), 31–55. I thank Sage Publications Ltd and the editor of *Social Studies of Science* for permission to draw upon my article 'Galileo and the embryos: religion and science in parliamentary debate over research on human embryos', 25 (1995), 499–532, copyright © 1995, Sage Publications Ltd. I thank Sage Publications Inc. and the editor of *Science, Technology and Human Values* for permission to draw upon the following of my articles: 'Women in the parliamentary debate over embryo research', 19 (1994), 5–22; and 'Frankenstein and the parliamentary debate over embryo research', 21 (1996), 157–76, copyright © 1994, 1996, Sage Publications Inc. I thank Daniel Callahan, President of the Hastings Center, for giving me permission to quote from the *Hastings Center Report*, January–February 1995, pages 39 and 42; Professor Dr Erwin Chargaff for permission to quote from 'Engineering a molecular nightmare', *Nature* 327 (21 May 1987), pages 199-200; the *Daily Mirror* for permission to quote two passages from the 'Baby Special' which appeared on 19 April 1990; Georgetown University Press for permission to quote from pages 13–14 of I. G. Barbour, 'Religion, values and science education', in D. Gosling and B. Musschenga (eds.), *Science Education and Ethical Values* (Georgetown University Press, 1985); HarperCollins Publishers for permission to quote from pages 124–5 of Andrew Kimbrell, *The Human Body Shop: The Engineering and Marketing of Life*, (HarperCollins, 1993); the Human Fertilization and Embryology Authority for permission to quote from page 4 of *Sex Selection: Public Consultation Document* (HFEA, 1993); *The Independent* Newspaper Publishing Plc for permission to quote from the issue published on 23 April 1990; The Labour Party for permission to quote from pages 100 and 102 of the *Report of the Annual Conference of the Labour Party 1985*; Macmillan

Magazines Ltd for permission to quote from *Nature* (Maxine Clark, 'Government stops Powell Bill', 314 (18 April 1985), page 573, and E. Chargaff, 'Engineering a molecular nightmare', 327 (21 May 1987), pages 199–200), copyright © 1985, 1987, Macmillan Magazines Ltd; *New Scientist* for permission to quote from 'Lords oppose embryo research', 104 (8 November 1984), page 6; Oxford University Press for permission to quote from pages 210–11 and 212 of L. Abse, 'The politics of in vitro fertilization in Britain', in S. Fishel and E. M. Symonds (eds.), *IVF: Past, Present, Future* (IRL Press, 1986); Random House UK Ltd for permission to quote from pages 101-2 of Robert Edwards and Patrick Steptoe, *A Matter of Life; The Story of a Medical Breakthrough* (Hutchinson, 1980), and from pages 62–6 of Robert Edwards, *Life Before Birth: Reflections on the Embryo Debate* (Hutchinson, 1989); Professor J. J. Scarisbrick for permission to quote from page 8 of *LIFE News*, No. 28 (Summer 1995); the editor, *Woman's Own*, for permission to quote from page 14 of the edition published on 26 August 1991; the editor, *Yorkshire Evening Press*, for permission to quote from the edition published on 21 March 1993. In addition, I thank Solo Syndication Ltd for selling me the right to quote from the editions of the *Evening Standard* published on 9 February 1990 and 19 April 1990, and from the editions of the *Daily Mail* published on 23 April 1990 and 16 July 1990.

Abbreviations

ALRA   Abortion Law Reform Association
BMA   British Medical Association
CORE   Comment on Reproductive Ethics
GIFT   gamete intra-fallopian transfer
HFEA   Human Fertilization and Embryology Authority
ILA   Interim Licensing Authority
IVF   *in vitro* fertilization
MRC   Medical Research Council
NIH   National Institutes of Health
SPUC   Society for the Protection of Unborn Children
VLA   Voluntary Licensing Authority

Introduction

In Britain, during the 1970s, the research team of Edwards, Steptoe and Purdy carried out a series of investigations into the *in vitro* fertilization (IVF) of human embryos which led, in 1978, to the birth of the first baby conceived outside a woman's body.[1] This achievement was widely publicized and quickly emulated by medical scientists around the world. By 1984, more than one hundred IVF clinics had been established in such scientifically developed countries as Australia, Austria, Belgium, Canada, Finland, France, Germany, Holland, Israel, Japan, Sweden, Switzerland and the United States.[2] In Britain, the number of IVF centres and the number of scientists engaged in research on human IVF embryos expanded rapidly. By the early 1990s, there were seventeen locations in the UK where projects in embryo research were under way and sixty-eight clinics employing IVF and related techniques for purposes of assisted human reproduction. In 1990, 1,443 women gave birth in Britain with the help of these techniques.[3] By the early 1990s, an estimated 20,000 'test-tube babies' had been born around the world, about one third of them in the USA.[4]

The immediate exploitation of major technical advances is normal in present-day medical science.[5] In this respect, the rapid growth of embryo research and assisted reproduction in Britain and elsewhere after the first IVF birth was not exceptional. In various other ways, however, the development of this area of scientific activity was unusual. This was particularly so in the UK.

In the first place, scientific research on human IVF embryos became the focus, in Britain, of intense public scrutiny which lasted throughout the greater part of the 1980s.[6] Secondly, although embryo research and assisted reproduction continued to expand during this period, research on human embryos was repeatedly attacked on moral grounds in Parliament and in other public settings. Despite enthusiastic support from the scientific community and from the medical profession, the continuation of embryo research was vigorously resisted by many ordinary people as well as by numerous special-interest groups. As a result, research of this kind came close to being banned by Act of Parliament and its future remained uncertain until the end of the decade.[7] Thirdly, even though research on human IVF embryos did eventually receive parliamentary approval, this approval was accompanied by a series of specific legislative restrictions on the scope of such research, by the establishment of elaborate mechanisms of external control over the conduct of those engaged in embryo research and by the introduction of severe penalties for infringement of the procedures set up to regulate the use of human embryos for purposes of scientific experimentation.[8]

The examination of the rights and wrongs of embryo research in Britain during the 1980s was highly unusual in the degree to which it subjected a particular branch of scientific inquiry to sustained, collective appraisal. The topic of research on human embryos generated a cumulative exchange of views which involved Members of Parliament, scientists, doctors, academics, the clergy, journalists, a wide range of interested organizations and pressure groups, and members of the population at large.[9] The public debate over embryo research led people to assess the morality of scientific research in its approach to such fundamental concerns as birth, death, disability and respect for human individuals. In the course of the debate, people's hopes and fears about this area of scientific investigation and their conflicting ideas about the place of the life sciences in present day society were publicly formed and displayed as they struggled to respond to the challenge posed by embryo research, and by the associated technology of controlled human reproduction.

In 1990, embryo research emerged from this long public review with recognition in law as a legitimate area of scientific inquiry. However, embryo research also emerged as a special scientific case; that is, as an area of experimental investigation which was generally regarded as permissible and as clinically valuable, but which was deemed to be sufficiently dangerous to require careful regulation from outside in order to ensure that it did not develop in ways inimical to the interests of the wider society.[10] In this study, I shall explore how scientific research on human IVF embryos came to be defined in Britain as a special case in need of special treatment and special safeguards.

In the chapters that follow, I shall show how public consideration of embryo research gave rise to controversy and to prolonged confrontation. I shall describe the dynamics of the struggle over embryo research, and the social and cultural origins of support for, and opposition to, such research.

I shall show how the battle over embryo research is reflected in the uneasy balance between endorsement and restriction that is a central feature of the legislation that eventually ensued. I shall also examine some of the cultural tensions that have been left behind by the public debate as well as the mechanisms of social control that were set up to deal with such tensions, and to guide the development of embryo research into the next century.

The first move towards sustained public debate over embryo research was taken in 1982, when the Department of Health and Social Security appointed a committee of inquiry, with the moral philosopher Mary Warnock in the chair, to 'examine the social, ethical and legal implications of recent, and potential developments in the field of assisted [human] reproduction'.[11] The report of the Warnock Committee was presented to, and discussed by, both Houses of Parliament in 1984. The Warnock Report dealt with a wide range of subjects; from the storage of artificially fertilized human ova to the administration of infertility services and the acceptability of commercial surrogacy.[12] The parliamentary debates that followed, however, as well as the wider public debate, came to be dominated by the question of whether or not research on human embryos was morally defensible and whether or not such research should be allowed to continue. This remained the most prominent, and by far the most controversial, topic of discussion arising from the Warnock Report. It was not finally resolved until Members of Parliament voted on the Government's Human Fertilization and Embryology Bill in 1990. In this study, the debate over embryo research will be my main concern. Other issues related to IVF and assisted reproduction will be considered only insofar as they bear on the public appraisal of such research.

The reception given to the Warnock Report in 1984 showed that many people, in Parliament and in society at large, were deeply disturbed to find that there was no law dealing with research on human embryos and no formal procedures whereby scientists could be made accountable for their use of human embryos. In response to these concerns, the Government promised, at the end of the first phase of parliamentary debate, that legislation would be introduced to cover activities of this kind. Henceforth, it was clear to all concerned that the future of embryo research would ultimately be decided by Parliament. As a result, public attention was drawn to the series of parliamentary debates held intermittently between 1984 and 1990 in which research on human embryos was the major topic.[13] These debates provided the central focus for the various pressure groups whose members wished to influence the legislative process. They were also the main stimulus for wider public discussion of embryo research.

Parliamentary appraisal of embryo research lasted for six years and included a period set aside explicitly for public consultation. There was, therefore, ample opportunity for the full range of public views and expert testimony concerning such research to find its way into the parliamentary forum. Consequently, in this study, I shall rely heavily on the verbatim record of parliamentary debate contained in Hansard. I shall use the parliamentary record as a lens through which to observe the struggle to determine how this area of British science would be allowed to develop.[14]

One obvious limitation of the formal parliamentary record is that it contains relatively little information about the lobbying, the private pacts or the informal discussions that occur whenever controversial issues are under consideration. Fortunately, these background negotiations were of particular interest to the scientific press and, to a lesser degree, to newspapers catering for a less specialized audience. Furthermore, the major lobbies concerned with embryo research made regular use of the press in their attempts to sway public opinion on this issue and to bring pressure to bear upon Members of Parliament. I have, therefore, compiled a body of additional material from the news sections of *Nature* and from the pages of *New Scientist* which documents at least some of these background activities.[15] I have also systematically examined a collection of newspaper cuttings covering the last six months of debate during which the Government Bill dealing with embryo research was passing through Parliament.[16] These three bodies of documentary material plus various official reports on matters related to embryo research[17] furnish the evidence for the findings to be presented in this study.

In the chapters that follow, I have tried to provide an accurate description of the struggle that took place as various groups of people with differing social and ideological commitments came together to determine the future of embryo research in the UK. I have tried faithfully to represent the views and actions of all those involved in this struggle, whether they were in favour of such research or opposed to its continuation. I have organized my discussion around a series of related themes which were regarded as important by participants and which were repeatedly addressed in the course of parliamentary debate. Thus, after reviewing the cultural context of the debate and summarizing the main sequence of events, I examine, in turn, the topics of political ideology, parliamentary lobbying, the mass media, gender, religion, science fiction, and the ethical regulation of embryo research. In each chapter, I compare and contrast participants' varied statements on a given topic in order to reveal the rhetorical structure of the debate and to build up an increasingly complex, multi-layered representation of the evolving contest. Although, in the last chapter, I look briefly at recent developments in the USA, the text concentrates primarily on the details of the debate in Britain. I have tried to use these details to construct a rich, yet clear and coherent, narrative which is accessible to a wide range of readers with quite different intellectual and practical interests.[18]

1

The background to the debate

Several of the major factors that determined the context in which the debate over embryo research took place can be traced back to the 1960s. This distinctive period in British public life also provides a useful point of contrast which helps to reveal more clearly why research involving human embryos became the focus of such vigorous controversy in the very different circumstances of the 1980s. In the first part of this chapter, I shall show how a combination of legislative reform and demographic change during the 1960s helped to create a potential demand for the reproductive techniques that grew out of such research in the 1970s. I shall then describe how the legislative reforms and the moral climate of the 1960s gave rise to a lasting political reaction which established the basis for organized opposition to embryo research in the 1980s.

The reform movement of the 1960s

In the second half of the 1960s, there was a wave of permissive legislation in Britain dealing with various matters of conscience. Because these matters lay outside the scope of the formal policies of the political parties, the new legislation was introduced by individual Members of Parliament in the form of Private Member's Bills. Between 1965 and 1969, five major Bills were passed which were intended to make the law less morally oppressive in relation to capital punishment, censorship of the theatre, homosexuality, divorce and abortion.[1] These legislative changes, apart from those dealing with capital punishment, were generally welcomed among the population at large. They were presented by their supporters as an expression of a natural need periodically to dismantle the antiquated morality left over from the past.[2]

This surge of legal reform, however, was not without its opponents. In

Parliament, these opponents were located mainly within the Conservative Party. Whereas most Labour and Liberal Members were in favour of the new legislation, Conservative Members were strongly inclined to be hostile.[3] The legislation was successfully enacted because the Labour Party was in power at this time, with a large parliamentary majority after the 1966 general election, and because the Labour Government was sympathetic both to the specific aims of the legislators and to the spirit of reform evident among Labour backbenchers.[4] The Abortion Act of 1967, although it had widespread public support and was finally approved in Parliament by a ratio of two to one,[5] was to become a particular focus of organized opposition in the years ahead and was, thereby, to influence the development of, and the public response to, research on human embryos.[6] It is necessary, therefore, to look more closely at the introduction of the new legislation on abortion.

Before the passage of the 1967 Act, few doctors in Britain were willing to undertake abortions openly. Thousands of women who wanted abortions were either refused permission or were too frightened even to raise the issue with their doctors.[7] At the same time, countless illegal 'back-street' abortions took place and fifty or more women died annually as a direct result of badly performed 'operations' carried out by untrained persons.[8] In these circumstances, a substantial number of people saw the existing legislation as excessively restrictive, as out of touch with contemporary notions of family planning and as damaging in its consequences.

The case for making legal abortion more accessible was presented with increasing urgency throughout the 1960s by a well-organized lobby, guided by the Abortion Law Reform Association (ALRA), which had recently been reinvigorated by an influx of young activists.[9] This lobby argued that the infant mortality rate had dropped to a level where it was no longer necessary for women to give birth at all costs in order to ensure that an adequate number of children survived to adulthood; that the spread of efficient contraceptive methods had encouraged and enabled women to take greater control of their own reproductive processes; that medical advances had made abortion a safe and painless operation when carried out in a proper clinical context; and that many ordinary, married women wanted to use, and should be allowed to use, abortion as a second line of defence against unwanted pregnancy.[10]

The introduction of the drug thalidomide into Britain in the early 1960s and the ensuing birth of a number of badly deformed children added weight to the arguments for reform of the abortion law. As a result of the public controversy over, and public condemnation of, thalidomide, abortion was taken out of the context of 'immorality and unmarried girls' and placed firmly in that of public health. With more and more sophisticated drugs becoming available, married women all over the country became concerned at the possibility of falling victim to a similar tragedy. Quite suddenly, in the wake of the thalidomide affair, the reformers were able to claim realistically that theirs was no longer a minority movement but an expression of general public opinion.[11]

It was in this atmosphere of widespread concern that the 1967 Abortion Act was introduced and given overwhelming support from the reformist Labour benches. The Act made abortion legal in situations where it was deemed to be necessary in order to preserve the physical or mental health of a pregnant woman or to avoid the birth of a seriously handicapped child. The Act allowed consideration of a pregnant woman's social environment and of the effect of a pregnancy on any existing children. Abortion was also held to be legal if it was safer for a woman than continuation of the pregnancy. During the 1970s, early abortion carried out by qualified medical personnel became increasingly safer than childbirth. This meant that the grounds for abortion under the Act were to become ever more inclusive.[12]

The 1967 Abortion Act greatly increased women's ability to use abortion, both inside and outside marriage, as a means of reproductive control. In 1969, the first full year after the Act came into effect, 50,000 legal abortions were notified in England and Wales for British women. By 1983, the number had risen to 127,000. In 1971, the proportion of abortions carried out on single women was 47 per cent; in 1983, this proportion had increased to 58 per cent.[13]

In the same year that the new law on abortion was enacted, the Cambridge embryologist Robert Edwards made contact with Patrick Steptoe, a gynaecologist and expert in laparoscopy at Oldham General Hospital. By the time that the provisions of the Act were fully in operation, these two men, in collaboration with their technical assistant Jean Purdy, had begun a joint programme of research and clinical practice and had succeeded in fertilizing human eggs outside a woman's body.[14] The long-term aim of Edwards and his colleagues was to develop reliable techniques of fertilization and reimplantation of fertilized ova which could be used to overcome certain kinds of human infertility. The idea of employing sophisticated methods of *in vitro* fertilization in this way had been present in scientific circles since the 1930s.[15] But it was not until the 1960s that, in view of recent scientific and technical advances, the clinical use of IVF on human subjects came to seem an imminent possibility.[16]

There is no evidence to suggest that Edwards, Steptoe and Purdy were in any way responding to, or influenced by, the arguments of the pro-abortion lobby during the 1960s in favour of women's reproductive rights. They seem, rather, to have been following up a newly created scientific opportunity to achieve a long-standing therapeutic goal. Nevertheless, the justification offered for their scientific activities closely paralleled the central moral claim of the pro-abortion movement. Whereas the pro-abortionists were asserting the right of fertile women to use science-based techniques to avoid bearing unwanted children, Edwards and his partners were seeking to develop techniques that would allow infertile people to assert the complementary right to bear children when they did want them.[17] Both the lobbyists and the scientists engaged in embryo research were strongly in favour of active intervention in the biological processes of human reproduction on the grounds that such intervention could improve the quality of family life and, in particular, that of women's lives.

During the 1970s, the legislative success of the pro-abortion lobby was to have unanticipated consequences which, in conjunction with underlying demographic trends, helped to increase the potential demand for a technological solution to the problem of childlessness within marriage. In the first place, the passage of the 1967 Abortion Act led to an immediate rise in the abortion rate. This, in turn, had the effect of reducing the supply of children available for adoption. In 1966, there were approximately 25,000 adoptions. The number had dropped to 13,000 by 1977 and continued to fall into the 1980s.[18] It seems that this decline was due partly to an increase in the use of contraception and to a growing unwillingness among single mothers to part with their children.[19] But the impact of the Abortion Act is evident in the fact that, within two years of its implementation, one third of the voluntary adoption agencies in Britain had closed.[20] The adoption of 'unwanted' children had been the customary solution to the problem of infertility within marriage. The 1967 Abortion Act contributed to making this solution less readily available than in the past.[21]

Both abortion and adoption have been associated historically with motherhood outside marriage. Until the 1960s, when attitudes began to soften, motherhood outside marriage was generally regarded in Britain as immoral. Because unmarried women were excluded from legitimate motherhood, most of them were obliged to remain infertile. Those who became pregnant and were unable or unwilling to marry were faced with a choice between illegitimacy, adoption and illegal abortion. This pattern of social demarcation and control operated within a society where, owing to differential rates of mortality and migration, there were many more women than men. In mid-Victorian England, roughly one woman in three was unmarried and, hence, morally required to remain sexually inactive. This demographic imbalance continued after the decimation of the male population in the First World War and did not finally disappear until the early 1960s.[22]

Involuntary infertility, therefore, was a major feature of British society before the 1960s. However, only that relatively small proportion of infertility that occurred among married people was seen to be a problem. The widespread infertility among women unable to marry was generally regarded as part of the natural order of things and as something to be accepted without comment.[23]

During the 1960s, the balance between men and women of marriageable age was finally re-established. As a result, the proportion of women able to marry increased considerably. Since the 1960s, 90 per cent of women have married by the age of thirty; and 90 per cent of men by the age of forty.[24] One major consequence of this dramatic increase in the proportion of married women in British society has been a significant social relocation of involuntary infertility from the unmarried to the married population.

Some clinicians and commentators have claimed that rates of biological infertility among British women have increased significantly since the 1960s as a consequence of environmental influences and of the growth of medical intervention in the reproductive processes occurring within women's bodies.[25] Other observers have rejected these claims or have judged them to be unproven.[26] However, even if rates of biological infertility have remained constant over this period, the increased frequency of marriage will have ensured that many fewer women will have been forced to endure the culturally invisible infertility previously required by spinsterhood, whilst many more women will have experienced infertility within marriage. This means that, since the 1960s, many more women than in the past will have been subject to the social pressure to reproduce that is brought to bear particularly on the female partner in an infertile marriage, and will have experienced the emotional turmoil induced by the failure to respond successfully to this pressure.[27] The difficulties facing such people have been increased by the sharp decline in the number of children available for adoption following the passage of the Abortion Act.

This was the situation that was beginning to take shape during the early 1970s as Edwards, Steptoe and Purdy began, for the first time, to reimplant human IVF embryos in a small number of infertile patients drawn from the gynaecological department of Oldham General Hospital.[28] Edwards and his partners were aware from their work in the hospital that the problem of infertility was being made worse by the fall in the adoption rate. They also sensed that, once people came to believe that a science-based remedy for infertility was available, the demand for their services would grow rapidly. Because they were dealing with married couples, Edwards and his colleagues were confident about their own moral position. They argued that their clients had an unquestionable right to become parents; and they presented their scientific and clinical activities as a benevolent attempt to satisfy their clients' rightful aspirations.

I had no doubts about the morals and ethics of our work. I accepted the right of our patients to found their family, to have their own children . . . It was a gift, the relationship of parent to a developing human being. And almost within our grasp was the possibility of passing on this gift to couples who had suffered years of child-lessness and frustration – who longed for children, who had indeed, as often as not, repeatedly undergone unsuccessful gynaecological operations in order to try to have children. The Declaration of Human Rights made by the United Nations includes the right to establish a family . . . Many of our patients had tried to adopt children repeatedly and without success. Moreover, adoption is likely to become even more difficult in the future with the spread of contraception and abortion, and with the rapid decline in the number of unwanted children. More and more couples would surely be pleading for the right to have their own child.[29]

Despite this strong moral defence, the programme of research and clinical development initiated by Edwards, Steptoe and Purdy in the late 1960s did not proceed without public opposition. In 1967, 1969, 1970 and 1971 there were brief bursts of criticism in the press and elsewhere. The main concern at this time was that the new techniques might produce abnormalities in the developing embryos or that they might be used to transfer embryos from one woman to another.[30] There was also a more general unease that this research might lead towards more radical forms of intervention in the bio-logical processes of human reproduction, such as selective breeding and eugenic control.[31] In 1971, a leading British embryologist publicly expressed the fear that Edwards and his colleagues were trying to go too far, too fast.[32]

At this stage, however, before the birth of the first test-tube baby, oppo-sition was sporadic and unorganized. Furthermore, as we have seen, certain major demographic processes were working to increase the number of people who would welcome Edwards's efforts to produce a science-based alternative to adoption. Unlike most of their critics, Edwards and his part-ners were directly in touch with such people and believed that there was widespread latent demand for the techniques of IVF. The birth of Louise Brown in 1978 immediately provoked renewed hostility to IVF and to embryo research.[33] But this widely publicized practical success also trans-formed the latent demand for a technological solution to the problem of childlessness into an active demand for the new techniques of assisted reproduction.[34]

The scientific and clinical investigations undertaken by Edwards and his colleagues during the 1970s were not linked in any direct way to the activi-ties or to the ideology of the pro-abortion movement. Nevertheless, by the early 1980s, as the number of test-tube babies started to grow, the arrival of IVF seemed to have added the final touches to the pro-abortionist programme of controlled reproduction in accordance with peoples' needs and preferences. It appeared likely, given increasing access to the new technology and a steady improvement in rates of successful implantation,[35] that infertility would soon be as well regulated as was fertility. This, at least, was the vision of Edwards and of many other practitioners in the realms of science and medicine.[36] However, this vision was not restricted to solving the problem of human infertility. As the new decade began, Edwards and others began to look towards a future in which research on human embryos would continue to open 'new horizons in human reproduction'[37] and to contribute to 'the benefit of humanity in directions which we do not apprehend today'.[38]

Edwards was aware, of course, that some people questioned the morality of his experimental procedures and that such people were not inclined to share his optimism about the long-term benefits of research involving human embryos. What he could not foresee at that juncture was that the reforms of the 1960s, and in particular the 1967 Abortion Act, had already generated a moral and political reaction which would nourish, in the years ahead, a sustained campaign of organized resistance to his vision of a world made better by continuing exploration in the field of embryo research.

The conservative backlash

The most successful parliamentary lobby during the 1960s in relation to moral issues was that organized by the Abortion Law Reform Association.[39] At that time, the ALRA had a clear legislative objective, a young, active membership and an extended network of influential contacts.[40] These features enabled the ALRA to sustain a lengthy campaign for legal reform in the media; and also in Parliament, by means of direct discussion with Members, by the circulation of Members on a regular basis and by arranging for the dispatch of letters from MPs' constituents.[41] The pro-abortion lobby was helped, as we have seen, by the political composition of the House of Commons, by the 'benevolent neutrality' of the Labour Government and by the public reaction following the tragic events brought about by the drug thalidomide. But it was also helped by the absence of organized opposition either within Parliament or in the wider society.[42] It was not until the Abortion Bill sponsored by the ALRA had received clear approval in the Commons on Second Reading in late 1966 that those opposed to major alteration to the law on abortion decided, in desperation, to co-ordinate their resistance by forming an equivalent body to the ALRA. The result of this decision was the creation, in January 1967, of the Society for the Protection of Unborn Children (SPUC).[43]

The SPUC was formed only six months before the decisive vote on the Abortion Bill took place. During this short period, opposition to the Bill increased substantially. Whereas the majority in favour on Second Reading had been 194, by Third Reading, in July 1967, it had fallen to 84.[44] The rapid progress made by the SPUC was insufficient to prevent enactment of the Bill. However, it seems to have encouraged those opposed to the new law to believe that their position was far from hopeless and that, over a longer time-span, it might be possible to obtain parliamentary approval for significant revision of the 1967 Act.

In 1970, a new organization called LIFE was formed, with the 'full knowledge and generous blessing of the founders of SPUC'.[45] LIFE's central objectives were to 'oppose all deliberate destruction of pre-born human life', and hence to 'strive for repeal of the [1967] Abortion Act rather than its mere amendment'.[46] At the same time, LIFE sought to provide counselling and practical help for women who were considering, or who had undergone, abortions. During the 1970s, these two closely linked organizations became increasingly well funded and efficiently administered. They also succeeded in attracting wide public support and became experienced in holding rallies and in bringing constituency pressure to bear on MPs of all parties.[47] Attacks on the Abortion Act began almost as soon as the Act had been passed. Between 1969 and 1982, eight attempts were made to enact legislation that would have restricted access to abortion more narrowly. All these attempts failed, but sometimes by very slender margins.[48]

Throughout the 1970s and 1980s, the SPUC and LIFE acted as the spearhead of organized opposition to the existing law on abortion. As the use of the phrase 'unborn children' implies, this opposition was based, in part, on the claim that the developing organism in the womb of a pregnant woman is a human being from the time of conception and is, accordingly, already a member of the human family with the same right to moral consideration as any other member.[49] It was argued, in the light of this claim, that the 1967 Abortion Act was immoral because it disregarded the rights of the unborn child, because it condemned to death countless innocent unborn children and because it involved, and encouraged, a denial of true parental responsibility. The existence of widespread approval of freely available abortion was acknowledged. But it was seen as one facet of a general moral decline which was thought to have accelerated out of control during the 1960s. Support for abortion, it was argued, grew out of the spread of sexual promiscuity and the erosion of traditional patterns of family life. The increased availability of abortion after the implementation of the Act, it was suggested, would reinforce this tendency towards moral degeneration. Thus opposition to the new law on abortion, in the 1970s, was seen by the lobbyists as part of a larger struggle in defence of a system of values and a way of life that was under threat.[50]

Concern over the supposed decline in moral standards since the 1960s has not been confined to the SPUC or to the other bodies, such as LIFE, that have made up the anti-abortion lobby. Numerous organizations critical of the overall moral climate in modern Britain, for example, the Responsible Society and the Moral Rearmament Association, were also established in the late 1960s and became increasingly active during the following decade. The members of these organizations were determined to restore to British society what they saw as the basic moral principles and the essential forms of conduct of the past. They were particularly disturbed by the changes in the patterns of family life that were revealed by the increasing rate of divorce, by the growing frequency of one-parent 'families' and by the increasing number of families in which both parents participated in paid employment outside the home.[51] They argued that the family was a fundamental social unit which exerted a determining influence on all other spheres of activity. They maintained that the present moral decline would be irreversible unless there was a wholesale return to the 'traditional nuclear family' in which the man was the breadwinner, in which the mother concentrated on her domestic duties and in which both parents acted as moral exemplars for their children.[52]

This pessimistic, backward-looking view of British society was especially prevalent during the 1970s among those who were members of, or were sympathetic towards the policies of, the Conservative Party.[53] Many of those who adopted this view held the Labour Party to be largely responsible for the supposed process of moral decay during the preceding decade. They insisted that restoration of the values and social practices destroyed under the corrosive influence of socialist doctrine would have to be a major objective when their own party returned to power. This position can be seen emerging as early as 1967 in a speech by a Conservative MP, at a meeting organized by the SPUC, who maintained that there was mounting evidence of depravity in the Labour Party. He claimed that Labour city councillors were advocating the establishment of legalized brothels, whilst Labour Members of Parliament were dismantling the laws that curbed homosexuality as well as making abortion available on demand. In his view, further development of this kind could be stopped only by the return of a Conservative government firmly committed to the moral principles on which the British way of life had previously been based.[54] In the words of another conservative moral activist, it had come to seem necessary, in order to regain the moral health of society, to reverse the 'rampant liberalism' of the 'immoral left'.[55]

The moral pressure groups formed in response to political and social change during the 1960s sought, throughout the 1970s, to make Conservative politicians more aware of the moral repercussions of their legislative activities and to encourage them to favour legislation that would promote a return to less permissive forms of conduct.[56] This strategy started to bear fruit after the Conservative victory in the general election of 1979 under the leadership of Margaret Thatcher. With the advent of the new Government, the rhetoric of British political life began to alter. Conservative politicians spoke with increasing firmness about the need for universal commitment to the long-established principles characteristic of British society at its best. The catchphrase 'a return to Victorian values' was introduced to convey, and to popularize, this message.[57] Particular attention was given to the reform of family life. A renewed emphasis on the importance of traditional motherhood was seen to be required. During the early 1980s, a Family Policy Group was set up to assist the Cabinet to find ways of restoring the 'heterosexual union, formed by marriage and nourished by children'[58] to its rightful place at the heart of British society.

These political developments coincided with the initial expansion in the clinical application of IVF. As the number of IVF pregnancies continued to rise, questions began to be asked, in Parliament and elsewhere, about the long-term implications of the new technology and of the research on human embryos with which it was associated.[59] It was coming to be generally accepted by this time that IVF and related techniques would enable more ordinary people to become parents. This, indeed, had been the justification for IVF and embryo research offered repeatedly by Edwards and his associates during the 1970s. The new technology of assisted reproduction could be seen, therefore, as making a positive contribution to the 're-establishment' of conventional family life. However, the control over human fertilization and over the distribution of fertilized ova conferred by the new techniques made possible the creation of family groupings and family relationships that had never before existed. Furthermore, it was coming to be realized by more of those involved in public life that the continuation of research in this area might eventually lead, in Edwards's words, 'in directions which we do not apprehend today'.[60] Unlike Edwards, many lay people saw this movement into the unknown as a potential threat to the predominance of the traditional family and to the values that form of family life was thought to express.

Concern over the destructive social impact that IVF and future reproductive techniques might have was felt particularly strongly in Conservative circles.[61] This concern is vividly conveyed in the statement below, by Lord Campbell of Alloway, which was made in the House of Lords on 9 July 1982:

LORD CAMPBELL My Lords, will my noble friend the Minister agree that without safeguards and serious study of safeguards, this new technique [IVF] could imperil the dignity of the human race, threaten the welfare of children, and destroy the sanctity of family life?

LORD LYELL My Lords, I am grateful to my noble friend. Indeed, what he says is entirely a strong possibility, and I am sure that his comments will be borne in mind by my right honourable friend [the Minister] in considering all the remarks that have been made in your Lordships' House today [on this topic].[62]

By the end of the month, the growing pressure for a thorough investigation of the social, legal and moral implications of the new techniques of assisted reproduction had led to the establishment of the Warnock Committee.[63]

The Warnock Committee consulted widely on matters related to assisted reproduction. After two years of deliberation, it distilled from these consultations sixty-four recommendations which were intended to be used as the basis for legislation.[64] The most important recommendation was that a new statutory authority should be created to monitor and to regulate both research and the provision of infertility services involving IVF and artificial insemination.[65] The committee concentrated on the use of the techniques of assisted reproduction in relation to the growing problem of infertility[66] and it emphasized that its members wished to uphold family values.[67] The report stated clearly that 'as a general rule it is better to be born into a two-parent family, with both father and mother'.[68] Nevertheless, the committee did not insist on formal union as a criterion of eligibility for access to assisted reproduction and it recommended that IVF should be made available to 'heterosexual couple[s] living together in a stable relationship, whether married or not'.[69] Thus, whilst the traditional family was reaffirmed in principle, the committee was willing to allow the new reproductive techniques to be used in ways that could be seen as encouraging illegitimate forms of parenthood.

The proposals with regard to research involving human embryos were equally cautious and considered, but equally likely to provoke opposition from the more conservative sectors of society. The creation and manipulation of IVF embryos, it was suggested, should become a criminal offence unless licensed by the proposed statutory authority. Donors of eggs and sperm would have to be consulted in advance about the use and disposal of any IVF embryos that were not implanted. The committee recommended that no IVF embryo should be kept alive longer than fourteen days and that it should be a criminal act to handle or to conduct research on an embryo that had lived beyond fourteen days.[70] In general terms, the committee proposed that embryo researchers should be firmly regulated by an independent body answerable to Parliament and narrowly restricted by law in their treatment of living human organisms. Nonetheless, within the specified constraints, the committee recommended that research on human embryos should be allowed to continue. It seemed unlikely that those who were particularly anxious about these new developments would be satisfied by the introduction of a time-limit which protected relatively advanced human embryos, but permitted scientists to use those that were less mature for experimental purposes.

The Warnock Report was presented to the Government in 1984 and was passed for discussion to a Parliament in which the Conservative Party had a large majority.[71] The fate of the Warnock proposals depended on their reception by the parliamentary representatives of that party. Among these representatives were many who were members of, or who had close contact with, the anti-abortion lobby. Although this lobby had been slow to comment on assisted reproduction, its members had gradually come to see direct links between the issues involved in the struggle over abortion and those arising from embryo research and the use of IVF. By 1984, the anti-abortionists had decided that assisted reproduction and abortion generated the same basic moral questions about the sanctity of human life, about our obligations to the unborn and about the nature of responsible parenthood. The anti-abortion lobby rejected the answers to these questions that were seen to be implicit in the major recommendations contained in the report of the Warnock Committee.[72]

Many members of the anti-abortion movement were concerned that the Warnock Report had failed to insist on the fundamental importance of marriage and that implementation of the proposal that IVF should be made available to unmarried people would further undermine the social position of legitimate families.[73] However, the main focus of their attack was the recommendations allowing the continuation of embryo research. Such research, maintained the anti-abortionists, was wrong in principle because, like abortion, it ignored the rights to life and protection enjoyed by all human beings whether they are born or unborn.[74] Parliamentary approval of embryo research, they claimed, would create a moral precedent and would open the way to other forms of even more repugnant experimentation as yet unimagined by the lay community. These arguments were submitted to the Warnock Committee. They may well have been taken into account by that committee. But they were not adopted as the moral basis for its proposals. Indeed, LIFE argued that the various elements of the pro-life case had been either caricatured or ignored in the Warnock Report.[75] As a result, the anti-abortionists decided that they had no option but to fight the committee's recommendations with the utmost vigour in the parliamentary setting.[76]

In the months leading up to the formal debates on the Warnock Report, the anti-abortion lobby worked hard to organize a display of parliamentary opinion which would be sufficiently impressive to persuade the Government to reject many of the main Warnock recommendations and, in particular, to repudiate embryo research. In the following passage, a Labour MP and enthusiastic supporter of embryo research describes how the anti-abortion lobby prepared systematically for the Warnock debates and managed to achieve its initial objective of ensuring that Warnock's proposals on this topic were strongly condemned by the great majority of speakers:

> SPUC works closely with a number of other organizations . . . All these organizations were poised waiting to attack the Warnock Report . . . SPUC was circulating briefing material to its members: it was immediately ready to publish and publicize comments attacking the Report on the day of its publication . . . When in October 1984 the Government put down a motion in the Lords to enable the Report to be debated, antagonistic feelings were apparent. The overwhelming majority of Peers who spoke were supporters of SPUC, probably echoing or slavishly following the briefs supplied to them . . . [A] month later when the Commons, at the instigation of the Government, debated the Report the House was packed with Conservative MPs eager to demonstrate to their local [anti-abortion] lobbyists their commitment to their cause . . . There were few Labour MPs present: those there to speak out for Warnock were the 'oldies', those of us who had fought in the sixties for divorce and homosexual and other reforms and for what we believed would be a more civilized society.[77]

We can see clearly from this quotation that the SPUC and its confederate organizations had developed into an efficient and powerful lobby. They had not, however, succeeded in changing the law on abortion. The recommendations of the Warnock Committee in favour of embryo research gave the anti-abortion lobby the opportunity to revitalize its activities and, perhaps, to attract additional members by focusing attention on the new topic of the destruction of 'unborn children' in scientific laboratories. By responding energetically against embryo research, the anti-abortionists sought to encourage widespread reconsideration of all those procedures that involved the destruction of human embryos or fetuses.[78]

There can be little doubt that organized opposition to embryo research was seen as the first step in a renewed campaign against abortion. But the expression of repugnance by the anti-abortionists at the use of living human embryos for experimental purposes was more than a tactical ploy. Embryo research was seen by them as intrinsically evil in the same way that abortion was seen as intrinsically evil. For the anti-abortionists, the arrival of embryo research marked one further stage in the moral decline that could be traced back to those legislative and moral innovations of the 1960s that were remembered with nostalgia by the Labour MP quoted above, but which were recalled with deep regret by his opponents. Furthermore, many people who were not members of the anti-abortion lobby were disturbed by the experimental use of potential human beings in pursuit of more scientific knowledge or in the development of new therapeutic techniques. Such objectives, they feared, could easily be employed as justification for ever more sinister forms of scientific activity.[79] As the parliamentary debates on the Warnock Report drew near, the lobbyists tried to play upon these feelings of unease and to shape them into co-ordinated opposition to the continuation of embryo research.

When the formal debates on the report began late in 1984, the SPUC and LIFE had helped to set the scene for a parliamentary confrontation very similar to that which had led to the formation of the SPUC seventeen years before. Although the topic now was embryo research rather than abortion, the anti-abortion lobby had made sure that the central moral issues to be examined would remain the same. This time, however, the balance of parliamentary power had been reversed. Parliament was dominated not by the Labour Party but by its Conservative adversaries. The parliamentary benches were filled this time, not with socialist reformers eager to remedy past mistakes and injustices, but with Conservative enthusiasts pledged to restore cherished patterns of conduct and moral principles that had been under pressure for most of the two preceding decades. Moreover, this time there was no equivalent to the ALRA to argue the case for unrestrained access to the fruits of scientific and medical advance. This time it was the conservative lobby that was well organized, virtually unopposed and in control of a large section of parliamentary opinion. As the Warnock debates began, the long sequence of action and reaction seemed to have turned full circle and the opponents of embryo research must have entered the parliamentary chambers with high hopes of obtaining a quick and decisive victory.

2

The sequence of parliamentary debate

The publication of the Warnock Report in July 1984 set in motion the sequence of parliamentary debate that formally established the legal status of embryo research in Britain.[1] The passage of the Human Fertilization and Embryology Act six years later brought this sequence to an end.[2] In the present chapter, I shall provide a simple, chronological account of the main phases of parliamentary debate and of the lobbying and public discussion that influenced parliamentary debate. In subsequent chapters, I shall examine in detail the major processes underlying this sequence of events.

1984: Warnock rejected

The main recommendations in the Warnock Report with regard to embryo research were that such research should be allowed to continue, but that it should be restricted in scope as well as monitored and controlled by a body outside the research community. External regulation of embryo research was justified by reference to the need to protect the human embryos used for experimental purposes, the need to safeguard the public interest and the need to allay widespread anxiety.[3] The report stated that the members of the committee were determined to prevent the 'frivolous or unnecessary' use of human embryos by those engaged in scientific research.[4]

Leading figures in embryo research responded angrily to this section of the report, repudiating the suggestion that scientists might undertake experiments on human embryos without careful consideration of their moral implications and rejecting the notion that researchers had to be held in check by the threat of criminal prosecution. Robert Edwards, for example, was quoted in *New Scientist* as saying: 'I deny the argument that [the] scientific impetus will necessarily lead to silly experiments. It would be unwise to jeopardize future advances by short-term recourse to the criminal law.'[5] In the accompanying article, it was reported that 'many scientists now fear that, in the light of the Warnock Committee's report, research on human embryos may be banned entirely. Much to the scientists' chagrin, the Committee appears to support the notion that all doctors are good and all scientists bad.'[6] In the same piece, another prominent researcher was quoted as claiming that 'the first part of the report is practical and sensible because it was based on at least 10 years of experience [with IVF]. When you come to the regulation of research it draws on science fiction and so is tinged with hysteria.'[7]

In *Nature*, although the anonymous editorial commentator was more subdued, the basic reaction was much the same. It was accepted that the use of new medical techniques sometimes had to be regulated and that the provision of IVF was similar in various respects to abortion and adoption, both of which were controlled by law. Research, however, was said to be 'quite a different kettle of fish'.[8] The fourteen-day time-limit on the use of embryos was denounced as arbitrary and the application of criminal sanctions beyond that limit was rejected as inappropriate and unnecessary. Scientific research, it was suggested, unlike most other human activities, cannot be regulated effectively because 'people cannot tell what they will find until they look'.[9] The editorial concluded that the sensible course of action would be to establish procedures of scientific self-regulation which would be open to public scrutiny and, thereby, responsive to legitimate public concern, but which would give researchers the freedom to continue to explore this exciting, important and potentially valuable area in a flexible and productive manner.

This largely negative response from the world of science prompted Mary Warnock to defend the conclusions on embryo research reached by her committee and to identify some of the underlying assumptions that had influenced its reasoning, but which had not been made fully explicit in the formal text.[10] She quickly made clear that she and her fellow committee members 'did not trust scientists and scientists alone to regulate themselves'.[11] She pointed out that reputable scientific journals had carried reports of likely advances in genetic manipulation, sex selection and so on, which would have social consequences well beyond the scientific community and which had given rise to justified public concern.[12] She insisted that the matters of public morality arising from such developments could not properly be decided solely by experts, especially by experts who were also interested parties, and that embryo research had to be seen to be conducted in a manner that was acceptable to the rest of society.[13] She maintained that external control of embryo research was essential because many ordinary lay people believed that scientists' overriding devotion to the pursuit of knowledge might sometimes lead them to pay insufficient attention to other values which non-scientists regarded as more fundamental.[14]

In the period following the publication of the report, Warnock tried to convince the scientific community and others broadly sympathetic to embryo research that there was widespread fear and distrust concerning such research in society at large; that it would be wrong as well as tactically inept simply to dismiss these feelings of anxiety as the product of scientific ignorance; and that something like the regulatory apparatus recommended in the Warnock Report was needed in order to provide reassurance for ordinary people. When Parliament met to discuss the report, it became evident that the safeguards and regulatory procedures intended by the Warnock Committee to allay ordinary people's suspicions of embryo research had not been sufficient to satisfy their parliamentary representatives; for most of those who spoke on this matter made it clear that their preference was for total prohibition.

The reaction in the Lords to the Warnock recommendations on embryo research was described in *New Scientist* as follows:

The House of Lords spoke out last week against any form of research on human embryos. In the first parliamentary debate on the recent Warnock Report on human fertilization and embryology, 18 out of the 24 peers who spoke opposed such research. Seven of them called for a two-year moratorium while the problems raised in the Report were thrashed out . . . Many speakers were concerned that permission to research on human embryos would lead to a devastating and irreversible erosion of society's moral values. The Bishop of Norwich said: 'I believe we should press the Government for a moratorium now, because the speed of research is going so fast that I believe we are moving into a Pandora's box which, when opened, will not be shut, and the opening of which will be not just for the moral hurt but for the family hurt of many people in many families in our country'.[15]

The debate in the Commons, three weeks later, was very similar. In this case, seven Members spoke in favour of the limited type of regulated research recommended by Warnock, whilst nineteen spoke against the continuation of embryo research in any form. As we would expect, in view of the preparation undertaken by the anti-abortion lobby, the basic arguments against embryo research were much the same as those used to condemn abortion; that is, that the early embryo is a person with full moral standing, that embryo research contravenes the rights of the experimental embryo and that failure to respect the embryo's rights is both a symptom of, and potentially a contributory factor in, the long-term decline of moral standards and proper family life. In accordance with Warnock's observations, this anti-abortion rhetoric was combined with a persistent questioning of scientists' capacity to control the consequences of their own experimental activities. All of these features are present in the following illustrative exchange taken from the opening debate in the Commons:

SIR GERARD VAUGHAN . . . My view is that . . . while the ovum and sperm have potential life, life begins at conception. It is unacceptable to bank fertilized ova and to experiment on human embryos, even for the first 14 days . . . Other issues flow from this work. What about animals and genetic manipulation? . . . There is the possibility of implanting fertilized ova into animals. The sheep-goat has already shown us the possibilities opening up of human–animal fusion; the mythological centaur begins to become an awful potential reality.

MR HUGH DYKES Is not one of the most insidious threats and risks to humanity that if, even under tightly controlled laboratory conditions, we allow so-called closely controlled experiments during the 14-day period, even the most stringent statutory authority could not ultimately control the nature of the experiment? Only the scientific technicians in charge of the experiments will be able to decide.

SIR GERARD VAUGHAN My hon. friend is absolutely right. I have paid particular interest to the sort of research undertaken, and whole areas of research now being considered are, I believe, wholly against the concept of any civilized society . . . If we do not act with authority, and rapidly, we shall find that scientific experiments intended for one purpose only have already rushed far ahead of what is acceptable . . . There is great urgency in this matter. The barriers should be set by this House, not by people outside. We, as a civilized Chamber and as a civilized society, should say that there is a limit to going too far down this road. Let us set it quickly and clearly.[16]

In both Houses, the few supporters of licensed research on the early human embryo were swept aside as the great majority of speakers rose to express their passionate indignation at the use of human individuals for experimental purposes and to press for the immediate cessation of these immoral activities.

By the end of 1984, the recommendations of the Warnock Committee with regard to embryo research had been shown to be unacceptable both to certain sectors of the scientific community and to a substantial number of parliamentary Members. It was clearly impossible, in these circumstances, for the Government to use these recommendations as the basis for legislation. Those Members who were most strongly opposed to embryo research insisted, however, that the issues raised by such research were too important to be left unresolved. They therefore urged the Government to abandon the Warnock proposals on research and to bring in a Bill that would express the view held by the great majority of Members that all research involving human embryos should be made illegal. The Minister for Health responded to this suggestion, at the end of the Commons debate, by maintaining that Parliament was too deeply divided over embryo research for the Government to take immediate legislative action along these lines.[17] It thus became clear that, if the opponents of embryo research wished to proceed further, they would have to demonstrate even more emphatically than in the opening debates that Parliament was not evenly divided on this issue, but was actively and overwhelmingly opposed to the continuation of embryo research.

The potential threat to embryo research implicit in this situation was noted by the editor of *Nature*: 'The danger . . . is that some MP will jump in with a Private Member's Bill drawn so emotively that nobody will dare oppose it'.[18] The idea of introducing a Private Member's Bill was attractive to the opponents of embryo research because, even if it was not enacted, it might give them the chance to force a vote and, thereby, if they were to achieve a large majority, to create further pressure on the Government to accede to their demand for a ban on all forms of embryo research. In the closing weeks of 1984, the agents of the anti-abortion lobby tried to make sure that a suitable Bill would be introduced early in the new year.[19]

1985: The threat of prohibition

None of the members of the lobby opposed to embryo research was highly placed in the ballot at the end of 1984 for the right to present a Private Member's Bill in the next parliamentary session. However, the lobby succeeded in gaining the co-operation of the Conservative ex-Minister Enoch Powell, who came near the top of the ballot and who was willing to collaborate in the introduction of a Bill to prohibit embryo research. Powell was not a member of the anti-abortion movement and had not previously been active in Parliament in relation to issues of this kind. He was opposed to embryo research, he insisted, not as a result of some prior ideological commitment, but simply because such research produced in him a deep feeling of moral repugnance and because he had discovered that this feeling was widely shared 'among all classes and callings and throughout the people of this country'.[20] The presentation of Powell's Unborn Children (Protection) Bill created the opportunity for a concerted attack on embryo research during the first half of 1985.

Powell's Bill was scheduled for full parliamentary debate at its Second Reading in mid-February. Several weeks before that date, the Medical Research Council (MRC) at last published its response to the Warnock Report. This document was also, in part, a reaction to the widespread opposition to embryo research that had become evident whilst the MRC was engaged in its lengthy deliberations and to the legislative vacuum that had arisen out of Parliament's failure to approve the Warnock recommen-dations.[21] The MRC proposed that this vacuum should be filled without further delay by the creation of an independent licensing agency which would supervise the development of embryo research on a voluntary basis until formal legislation was enacted based on the Warnock Report. The MRC promised to help set up such an agency in the near future. Doubts were expressed in the MRC report about the fourteen-day limit on research recommended by Warnock. It was argued that, because embryos may grow at different rates in different circumstances, it would be more satisfactory to define the limit on research in terms of the stage of embryonic growth. Nevertheless, the secretary of the MRC made clear that the proposed vol-untary body would comply with the procedures specified in the Warnock Report and would 'not permit scientists to research with or handle embryos that are older than 14 days'.[22]

In *Nature*, editorial discussion of the MRC report was combined with assessment of the threat posed by Powell's Bill. The latter was dismissed as 'half-baked legislation'. However, it was seen as distinctly possible that Parliament would be 'stampeded into over-hasty' enactment of this legis-lation – which would persist 'as law until some future Government has the political courage to take on the alliance of interests opposed to novel practices in human embryology'.[23] It was suggested that the present Government should prevent this from happening by adopting the proposal originating in the Warnock Report, and recently endorsed by the MRC, that a licensing authority for research on human embryos should be estab-lished.

This authority, it was argued, would need to be 'backed by a legal requirement that would-be innovators should disclose their plans and wait for them to be approved'. The authority's main task would be to consider on its merits any scientific investigation involving human embryos, includ-ing experiments that Warnock would have rejected on principle, and to issue licences for those projects deemed to be acceptable. Action of this kind, it was asserted, 'is the only way forward that makes sense. And that could be done quickly, perhaps even by next Friday'.[24] The suggestion that it might be possible to outflank the imminent parliamentary attack on embryo research by setting up a licensing authority in less than a week was totally unrealistic; perhaps 'half-baked' would be a more appropriate description. It gives the impression that there was a mood approaching panic in the editorial office of *Nature* at the prospect of the forthcoming debate in the House of Commons.

The debate over the Unborn Children (Protection) Bill in February 1985 proved to be a resounding victory for the opponents of embryo research and confirmed the worst fears of the scientific community. The Bill was designed to ensure that the clinical application of IVF would be controlled more closely than in the past and to prevent any use of IVF embryos for experimental purposes or, indeed, 'in any other way or for any other purpose except to enable a woman to bear a child'.[25] The distribution of speakers was actually more evenly balanced than in the two preceding debates; with thirteen Members speaking for, and eleven against, the prohibition of embryo research. But the vote of two hundred and thirty-eight to sixty-six in favour of Powell's Bill[26] revealed overwhelming parliamentary opposition to the continuation of research involving human embryos. The pragmatic view of the pro-research minority that embryo research should be allowed to continue in order that people might enjoy its therapeutic benefits was firmly rejected. The great majority of Members seem to have been more moved by the argument eloquently expressed by one of the leading figures in the campaign against abortion that 'our responsibility is to proclaim the old values of the dignity and uniqueness of all human life . . . and to erect barriers beyond which the tyrannies of scientific technique shall not pass'.[27]

The scientific community had expected the House of Commons to approve Powell's Bill on Second Reading. Nonetheless, there seems to have been considerable surprise at the size of the majority. The scientific and medical establishment was described in *New Scientist* as being 'shocked' at the outcome of the debate. Researchers were reported as finding it 'incredible' that some of their activities might soon become criminal offences. The MRC was said to be 'furious at the attempt to sabotage much of its work in this area'.[28] Antagonism towards embryo research among MPs was attributed by an MRC official to their ignorance of scientific matters.[29] The moral position of the critics of embryo research was parodied in *Nature* as the simplistic view 'that embryos are people, and that killing people is wrong'.[30]

At the same time, however, there was a more thoughtful, and a more politically astute, response from within the world of science to the situation created by the visible supremacy of the anti-research lobby. Three weeks after the vote on Powell's Bill, *Nature*'s editorial voice tried to view embryo research from the perspective of ordinary people with no scientific background. The journal's readers were asked to consider why such people should regard scientific research as sacrosanct, 'especially when it flatly conflicts with what seems to be an absolute moral principle'.[31] The struggle on behalf of embryo research, it was suggested, must begin with acceptance of the fact that all research has to be justified to the satisfaction of the lay community and its parliamentary representatives. The editor pointed out that the substantial body of parliamentary opinion opposed to embryo research would not simply melt away. The advocates of such research were urged to face up to the task of persuading MPs, and the population at large, 'that some other course of action than Mr Powell's Bill will meet their need'.[32] This could best be done, the editor maintained, by making sure that people properly understood what would be lost by the prohibition of research on human embryos.

In the next issue of *Nature*, either by chance or by design, this strategy was put into operation in an article that attempted to show how enactment of Powell's Bill would prevent specific advances in the treatment of infertility, in the development of new contraceptive techniques and in the control of various genetic disorders. The article ended by confronting those who were opposed both to abortion and to embryo research with the argument that research on early embryos would lead to a reduction in the number of spontaneous abortions as well as in the number of abortions induced on genetic grounds and would, therefore, if it was allowed to continue, have the morally welcome effect of making recourse to abortion significantly less frequent.[33] Thus, within weeks of the vote in support of Powell's Bill, there were clear signs in *Nature* of the emergence of a more active approach within the scientific community to the struggle on behalf of embryo research.

This positive reaction to the disastrous Second Reading of Powell's Bill was not confined to the scientists. Many lay people who supported embryo research began to present their views more vigorously in the media and in the political arena. The massive defeat in Parliament seems to have convinced both practitioners and supporters of embryo research that they needed to try much harder, as *Nature* had recommended, to influence public opinion. In the words of one, evidently partisan, Member of Parliament:

The medical and scientific community became alarmed and those who came to sympathetic MPs for advice were quickly instructed that . . . they must learn to defend themselves. There were not a few who learned with speed to shed their political innocence and come out of the laboratory and the gynaecology wards to join the battle in public debate with great administrative and presentational skills. The Medical Research Council recanted and threw its full weight behind Warnock. The feminist movements and the traditional pro-abortionist lobbies infuriated by the coup of their old anti-abortionist enemies entered the fray with relish . . . Meantime Lady Warnock and many on her Committee, in the press and on the media penetratingly explained the issues which the fundamentalists had obfuscated.[34]

As the time approached for the decisive, final report stage of Powell's Bill, resistance to the anti-research lobby became more vigorous and the verbal battle over embryo research became more heated. Although it seemed most unlikely that the balance of parliamentary opinion would be significantly altered in the course of a few weeks by the processes of public debate, formal parliamentary approval of the Unborn Children (Protection) Bill was by no means inevitable. For Powell's Bill was a Private Member's Bill and stood little chance of being enacted unless the Government were willing to grant certain procedural concessions. Powell's supporters argued that the Government should deal sympathetically with the Bill in view of the huge majority it had achieved at Second Reading. But this argument was ignored by the Government and, three weeks before the final session was due, it was announced that no extra time for debate would be provided. As a result, those opposed to the Bill, despite being greatly outnumbered, were easily able to talk the Bill out of time[35] and, thereby, to enable those engaged in embryo research and in the clinical application of IVF to continue as before.

The opponents of embryo research, like the scientists some months earlier, were reported to be furious at this set-back.[36] They did not, however, admit defeat. Within a few weeks, they made unexpected use of House of Commons rules in an attempt to reintroduce Powell's Bill for further discussion. This attempt was blocked only by means of equally skilled procedural manoeuvring on the part of MPs favourable to embryo research.[37] Undeterred by this failure, the members of the anti-research lobby turned their attention once again to the annual ballot for Private Member's Bills.[38] At this point, it became clear that the central group controlling much of the parliamentary opposition to embryo research was determined to persevere with a long-term campaign of action along the lines employed previously in relation to the law on abortion. The implication for those who were fighting for the continuation of research on human embryos became equally clear; namely, that they were unlikely to succeed unless they established an organized lobby of their own to match that of their adversaries.

Accordingly, in November 1985, an association called Progress was formed, under the joint leadership of scientists, physicians and parliamentarians. This group's first act was to launch a campaign at the House of Commons intended to increase public understanding of, and support for, embryo research.[39] At the same time, the Voluntary Licensing Authority (VLA), which had been set up by the Medical Research Council and the Royal Society of Obstetricians and Gynaecologists whilst the Powell Bill was under consideration, began to issue the first licences for externally supervised research on IVF embryos.[40] By the end of 1985, the researchers, the medical and scientific establishment and the lay supporters of embryo research had at last begun to create the basis for organized opposition to the critics of embryo research.

In response to the initial ascendancy of these critics and to the likelihood of further private legislation modelled on the Powell Bill, the defenders of embryo research agreed to work together in support of the main recommendations contained in the Warnock Report. As a result, the movement in favour of embryo research became more capable of sustained and co-ordinated political action. There can be no doubt that the opponents of such research were still dominant in Parliament and that they had considerable backing among the general public. Nevertheless, the response of the pro-researchers during 1985 to the threat of prohibition had ensured that the balance of power between the two sides would be less unequal in future. Furthermore, one item in *Nature* earlier in the year had seemed to suggest that people's views about embryo research might be changed, as their views about abortion had been changed in the 1960s, if a sufficiently strong link could be established between research on human embryos and increased control over the incidence of genetic disability.

A Marplan opinion poll published in Britain this week . . . reveals that 32 per cent of adults are in favour of embryo research, 41% are against and 27 % 'don't know'. Nearly half of the opponents changed their minds when asked if they would favour research if it would help to eliminate genetic diseases, resulting in a total of 51 per cent in favour of research.[41]

In the press campaign organized by Progress, attention was drawn to the possibility that embryo research might lead eventually to the development of techniques for screening out embryos with genetic defects.

1986-7: Parliamentary manoeuvres and legislative delay

The anti-research lobby continued its efforts during 1986, but with less success than in the opening phase of parliamentary activity. At the time of the first debate over Powell's Bill, LIFE had delivered to Parliament a petition for the protection of the human embryo with two million signatures. In January 1986, a similar petition was presented to the House of Commons. But, on this occasion, there were only 203 signatures from the 'national officers and chairmen of LIFE's regions and groups'.[42] This petition requested that the House take immediate steps to enact legislation to protect 'the human embryo from any practices which violate his/her dignity or right to life'.[43] Its purpose was to solicit renewed support for the Unborn Children (Protection) Bill which had been submitted to the Commons once more, this time by Ken Hargreaves. The Bill was opposed by two small petitions which urged the House to vote against Mr Hargreaves's Bill. In the event, there was insufficient time for the Bill to be discussed and no vote was possible.[44]

In October 1986, Hargreaves took advantage of the Commons' elaborate procedures to present the Bill yet again in the form of a 'ten-minute Bill'. Hargreaves used the short time available to castigate his opponents for ignoring the fact that 'the human embryo is undeniably a member of the human species' and to exhort the House to prohibit by law the use of such embryos in harmful experiments. He criticized the supporters of embryo research for painting a misleadingly 'rosy picture of the benefits for society if only we allowed scientists freedom', and condemned the scientists, in turn, for inventing the 'Humpty Dumpty word "pre-embryo"' to diminish the status of human individuals at their earliest stage of development. He claimed that there was still a huge majority in Parliament and elsewhere in favour of the Unborn Children (Protection) Bill and he accused the pro-researchers of trying, undemocratically, to prevent the views of the population at large from being heard in Parliament. Thus, this brief debate was not a mere formality, he argued, but a crucial opportunity to record a vote that would 'show the British public that the majority in this House is concerned to see something done to protect the human embryo'.[45]

The reply came from Peter Thurnham, who had presented the petitions in January denouncing the Unborn Children (Protection) Bill. Thurnham rejected Hargreaves's assessment of the human embryo as inconsistent with medical opinion. He claimed that the recommendations of the Warnock Report in favour of controlled embryo research had already been adopted in Australia, Japan and the US, and that the Voluntary Licensing Authority was 'the envy of the world'. If Mr Hargreaves's Bill were to be enacted, he suggested, British scientists would flee abroad. As a result, there would be less research in the UK devoted to improving IVF success rates and to preventing the transmission of genetic disease. Fortunately, in Thurnham's view, enactment of the Bill was most unlikely because opposition to embryo research was confined to a 'vociferous minority' that 'flies in the face of majority public opinion which has been expressed clearly in favour of human embryo research aimed at prevention of congenital handicap'. Thurnham called upon his fellow parliamentarians to show their support for embryo research by rejecting the Bill and by agreeing to wait patiently for appropriate Government legislation based on the Warnock Report.[46]

Thurnham's call was unsuccessful. The Unborn Children (Protection) Bill was approved by the House of Commons for a second time by 229 votes to 129. This result provided considerable justification for Hargreaves's claim that a clear majority of Members, or at least of those Members actively interested in the issue, was still in favour of banning embryo research. Yet Thurnham could derive some comfort from these figures. For the vote against research had not increased, whilst the number of MPs voting against the Bill had doubled from 66 to 129. It was, of course, impossible for either side to interpret the changing pattern of voting with confidence in a situation where half the House did not participate and where there was no real possibility of enactment flowing from the vote. Nevertheless, although this display of parliamentary strength had been engineered by the critics of embryo research, it may well have given greater encouragement to Thurnham and his pro-research companions. For the latter could reasonably infer that they had not lost ground in the Commons since the vote on Mr Powell's Bill and that their position might actually have improved substantially.[47]

Outside Parliament, the campaign on behalf of embryo research was continuing to expand, but was also experiencing difficulties with its scientific constituents. Both Progress and the Voluntary Licensing Authority had decided to replace the word 'embryo' with 'pre-embryo' when referring to the human organism during the period of approximately two weeks between fertilization and the emergence of the first structural features. This new terminology was intended to help undermine their opponents' use of the phrase 'unborn children' and to convey to lay people that the potential subjects of laboratory experiment were not even proper human embryos.[48] Many of those active within the world of science, however, were unhappy with what they saw as a conscious and misleading manipulation of words to further the interests of the pro-research lobby.[49] They regarded the introduction of this ostensibly technical term into the public debate as an attempt to hide what were really moral and political judgments behind an illusion of scientific objectivity. Some scientists were led to challenge, not only the campaigners' use of words, but also the basic claim about the nature of the early embryo which underpinned the moral argument that embryo research was permissible in principle.

The 'pre-embryo' is a designation that appears to me entirely unjustified. I fear that it has merely an alibi function. The life of the embryo begins with the fertilized egg in which all the potentialities of the organism reside. The attempt to determine, by scientific means, the stage at which what for times immemorial had been called the human soul makes its appearance, is ridiculous. The setting of a calendar date serves only as a permit for the performance of experiments that normal reverence before human life would have outlawed: experiments that until a few years ago would, in fact, have been unthinkable.[50]

This wholly negative view of the morality of embryo research was not widely shared within the scientific community. But rejection of the term 'pre-embryo' was widespread. The editor of *Nature* called the word a 'cop-out' and suggested that it should be banned.[51] *New Scientist* had declared earlier that the new word would fool no one and that critics of embryo research would be able to cite this dubious neologism to reinforce people's doubts and fears about scientists' intentions.[52] As we have seen, this is precisely what Hargreaves tried to do when he described 'pre-embryo' disparagingly in the course of parliamentary debate as a 'Humpty Dumpty word'. Thus, although it was possible for the supporters of embryo research to maintain, during this period, that their campaign was having a positive impact in Parliament, it was clear that some of the rhetoric employed in that campaign was creating open divisions within the scientific community which must have strengthened the confidence of their opponents.

In December 1986, whilst these terminological disputes continued to simmer in the scientific press, the Government initiated the next phase in the legislative process by issuing a discussion paper reviewing the full set of recommendations contained in the Warnock Report.[53] This paper was distributed mainly to 'recognized professional bodies' with the aim of generating further consultation on these issues before the Department of Health and Social Security began to draft formal legislation in the latter half of 1987.[54] The document distinguished between those recommendations in the Warnock Report where a broad measure of agreement was likely and those that were still contentious. The use of human embryos for research was identified as the most difficult issue and as a matter that required special legislative treatment. It was proposed that alternative clauses should be provided which would allow Members of Parliament to vote on the future of embryo research according to their consciences rather than along party political lines. The paper envisaged that one clause would prohibit research on IVF embryos, whilst the other would permit embryo research under the conditions specified in the Warnock Report.

The distribution of this consultative document was widely condemned as unnecessary. A spokeswoman for the SPUC denounced it as 'a blatant delaying tactic' on the part of a morally confused Government and as 'nothing but a rehash of Warnock'. Her opposite number from Progress also criticized the Government for their failure to act decisively, but added the optimistic comment that the delay would help the supporters of embryo research because public opinion was swinging in their favour.[55] This return to consultation with representatives of the wider community after two-and-a-half years of parliamentary negotiation had the effect of bringing parliamentary activity on embryo research to a halt throughout the whole of 1987, whilst both sides waited for the Government to come back with its final legislative proposals. It was clear, nonetheless, that this was no more than a temporary cessation of hostilities. For the Government's apparent preference for a free parliamentary vote on this topic seemed to indicate that the fate of embryo research would have to be decided, sooner or later, by direct confrontation in Parliament between its supporters and its opponents.

1988-9: Growing pressure for Government legislation

The Government's consultative exercise took a whole year to complete. It did not, however, produce a Bill, but merely a White Paper, or policy document, outlining a framework for legislation. This document required further parliamentary appraisal before the final, decisive, step would be taken.[56] The White Paper inevitably followed the recommendations of the Warnock Report on embryo research fairly closely. It was proposed to replace the Voluntary Licensing Authority with a Statutory Licensing Authority to regulate infertility treatment and, if it were to be permitted, embryo research. Similarly, if such research were to be allowed, use of human embryos beyond fourteen days after fertilization or after the appearance of the primitive streak was to be forbidden under pain of imprisonment. But the White Paper did not endorse the Warnock recommendation in favour of the continuation of embryo research. Instead, it proposed that the eventual Bill would use the device of alternative clauses on embryo research to enable Members of Parliament to decide this issue according to their personal judgment.

The White Paper also placed a series of additional restrictions on embryo research in relation to genetic engineering and related activities. The Warnock Report had devoted only two paragraphs explicitly to the prevention of genetic defects and to public anxiety about the possible manipulation by scientists of human beings' genetic endowment. It was argued by the committee that such techniques of genetic control were 'purely speculative' and that improper developments in this area would be prevented by the ordinary procedures involved in licensing and monitoring embryo research.[57] The White Paper, in contrast, emphasized that 'one of the greatest causes of public disquiet has been the perceived possibility that newly developed techniques will allow the artificial creation of human beings with certain predetermined characteristics through modification of an early embryo's genetic structure'.[58] The White Paper promised that, although the prospects for achieving these genetic techniques were remote, the proposed Bill would explicitly forbid research of this kind. The same reasoning was used to justify the introduction of clauses prohibiting the cloning of human cells and the transfer of human embryos to another species.[59]

The new restrictions upon embryo research included in the White Paper were, in part, a response to the activities of the anti-research lobby, which had not only given forceful expression to public anxiety about genetic engineering, but had also sought to foster such anxiety. These concessions, however, did not make the parliamentary opponents of embryo research any less critical of the White Paper. Once again, they denounced the Government's proposals as no more than a repetition of Warnock. The new prohibitions were dismissed as relatively minor adjustments in a document that had been written from a perspective covertly favourable to embryo research.[60]

The supporters of embryo research were equally critical of the White Paper, but for rather different reasons. Both *New Scientist* and *Nature* drew attention to the way in which the national newspapers had concentrated on the new clauses dealing with genetic engineering and had depicted the Government in the idiom of science fiction as acting to prevent recalcitrant scientists from carrying out horrific experiments. *Nature* reported despairingly that the *Sun* had even printed a still from the film *Frankenstein*.[61] The scientific press concluded that the attempt by Government to reduce public unease about embryo research had been represented to the population at large in a way that could only have made people more worried than before and, therefore, that the publication of the White Paper had probably led inadvertently to a decline in public approval of embryo research.

The scientific press also contained numerous expressions by scientists of disappointment that the Government had chosen not to introduce legislation that would guarantee the continuation of embryo research, 'but instead to take pot luck with a free vote in the House of Commons'.[62] It was assumed that a Government Bill would follow fairly quickly after parliamentary discussion of the White Paper and that Members would almost certainly use their free vote to make embryo research illegal. In much the same way that many parliamentarians were distrustful of scientists and of scientists' experimental methods, many members of the scientific community were distrustful of politicians and of the parliamentary process. As *Nature*'s editor put it: 'This is, after all, the Parliament that required that men with red flags should walk in front of the early motor cars.'[63] The House of Commons was viewed as particularly unreliable. It was suggested that its Members tended to vote in relation to contentious matters, not on the merits of the contending arguments, but to please their most strident constituents.[64] In addition, it was claimed that 'there are many people in the House of Commons eager for a chance to rattle the threat that devilish experiments with human embryos are around the corner to support the case that abortion should be forbidden'.[65] The White Paper was worrying for many scientists because it made clear that the final decision on embryo research would be made by people who were thought to have little sympathy for, or understanding of, the world of science.

As the parliamentary debates on the White Paper approached, the scientific press was in pessimistic mood. Nevertheless, neither *Nature* nor *New Scientist* was willing to give up hope. The public advocates of embryo research were urged to increase their participation in the media still further and to renew their efforts to put across the basic message that, in *Nature*'s words, 'the social benefits of continuing research would be considerable'.[66] *New Scientist* was more specific. A practitioner was quoted who maintained that 'research on human embryos is about alleviating the suffering of families at risk of [genetic] diseases such as Lesch Nyhan and muscular dystrophy'.[67] Thus, for *New Scientist*, the task ahead was to make enough MPs understand that a ban on embryo research would stop further advances in the diagnosis of genetic disease and would, thereby, lead to the continuation of much avoidable human suffering.

The formal debates on the White Paper in January and February 1988 turned out to be more favourable to embryo research than the scientific press had expected. The overall balance of parliamentary opinion remained unclear because there was no vote in either House. Nevertheless, in the Lords, thirteen speakers expressed firm support for the continuation of such research under the conditions specified in the White Paper, whilst only seven Members spoke wholly against research on human embryos. Even in the Commons, there was a small majority in favour of embryo research, with ten speakers for, and eight speakers against, its continuation. Thus, for the first time, the case in favour of embryo reseach was ascendant in parliamentary debate. Furthermore, there were clear signs that the points made by, and even the terminology used by, Progress were being adopted by parliamentarians. Some of them, for example, were beginning to refer, not to embryo research, but to pre-embryo research. Similarly, Members were much more familiar than in the past with those potential benefits of embryo research on which its publicists had placed such stress.

In the course of these debates, the opponents of embryo research vigorously attacked the press campaign organized by Progress as well as the research itself. But many speakers agreed with Progress that research involving early human embryos was not intrinsically immoral and that it should be allowed to continue, under close supervision, in order to bring to realization its potential therapeutic benefits. These speakers emphasized that there was a 'compelling and urgent need for everything possible to be done to advance research aimed at preventing congenital handicap'.[68] Other benefits of embryo research were regularly mentioned in both debates. But the possibility that such research might significantly reduce the level of genetic disease was treated as a particularly powerful argument in its favour.

Six weeks after the second of these debates, in March 1988, the members of the anti-research lobby at Westminster began a new campaign to strengthen opposition to embryo research. It seems likely that this was a reaction to their disappointing performance in the debates on the White Paper and an attempt to reverse the apparent growth in parliamentary support for embryo research. A report was presented entitled *Upholding Human Dignity: Ethical Alternatives to Embryo Research.* Its central themes were that embryo research was immoral, that it would lead to ever more radical forms of scientific intervention in the biological processes of human reproduction and that other, morally acceptable, kinds of research could be used more effectively to improve the treatment of human infertility and to deal with the problems of genetic disease.[69]

This campaign was launched on the clear understanding that the Government's Bill was imminent and that parliamentary opposition to embryo research had to be maintained in readiness for the final confrontation. The supporters of embryo research also expected that, now that the Government's legislative framework had been considered by Parliament, a Bill based on that framework would be introduced during the next parliamentary session beginning in November 1988.[70] In September, however, the MP and parliamentary columnist of the *New Scientist*, Tam Dalyell, reported that 'the widely anticipated bill concerning research on embryos is likely to vanish from the Queen's speech in November. It is not just a matter of pressure on the legislative timetable of Parliament. The truth is that it is a hot potato, which the Government's business managers see no pressing reason to bring to the fore.'[71] Two months later, Dalyell's prophecy was shown to have been correct.

Many of those actively involved in the debate over embryo research believed, of course, that the need for action was urgent. Many were inclined to the view that there must be some ulterior motive behind the Government's refusal to act after four-and-a-half years of consultation, formal appraisal and parliamentary discussion. This was particularly true of those who wished to bring embryo research to a stop. They found it difficult to understand why a Government that claimed to be neutral with regard to embryo research could not simply allow Parliament to decide this matter by means of open debate followed by a free vote on the alternative clauses. More than fifty MPs lodged complaints over the delay. The Archbishop of Westminster wrote to the Government, on behalf of those opposed to embryo research, to express dismay that no Bill was forthcoming.[72] At the same time, the chair of the Voluntary Licensing Authority complained that, when her authority had been set up in 1985, its members had been told that it would operate for one year only. She reported that it had been decided to change its name to the Interim Licensing Authority (ILA) partly as a reminder to the Government that a statutory body must soon be established.[73]

In response to these frustrating circumstances, the anti-research lobby decided to present for discussion in the Lords another Private Member's Bill closely based on the Unborn Children (Protection) Bill. The Duke of Norfolk stated in his introductory speech that the purpose of the Bill was to spur the Government into action in order to bring to an end a situation where 'many of us feel that unethical deeds are taking hold in parts of the medical profession'.[74] In reply, Lord Houghton quoted from a memorandum said to have been signed by the Duke, in which it was stated that the Government were thought to be delaying their own bill in order to allow parliamentary opinion time to move further in favour of embryo research and that the 'pro-life' lobby had to act immediately to demonstrate that there was still considerable strength of feeling against such research in the Upper House. In the light of this memorandum, Lord Houghton ridiculed the reintroduction of Powell's Bill as little more than an attempt by the Duke to 'whip up his pro-life friends' in order to dispel the poor impression created by their resounding defeat in the debate on the White Paper.[75]

The debate in the Lords over the Unborn Children (Protection) Bill was staged by the anti-research lobby, at least in part, to show that, although embryo research may have become more popular in the Upper House over the years, there were many who remained deeply opposed to its continuation.[76] At the same time, the debate had a wider significance in that it helped to make clear to both sides that further parliamentary maneouvring on this subject was pointless, that all the prerequisites for comprehensive legislation were in place and, therefore, that the Government should delay no longer. Thus Lord Houghton summarized the outcome of this debate, and indeed of this phase of parliamentary negotiation, with the following call for action: 'The message from the House tonight is for the Government to produce this legislation.'[77]

1989-90: Victory and defeat

By November 1989, it was known that the Government were, at last, about to introduce their own Bill dealing with embryo research and use of the techniques of assisted reproduction. It was also known that the forthcoming Bill would follow closely the proposals contained in the White Paper. Although it was clear that the promise concerning the provision of alternative clauses on embryo research would be honoured in the Bill, it seems that rumours were circulating to suggest that the Government were secretly in favour of the option that would allow the continuation of research involving human embryos. The Secretary of State for Health, Kenneth Clarke, declared publicly that this accusation was untrue. 'The Government does not take a collective view,' he stated, 'we believe that such matters should be left to the conscience of the individual Member.'[78] At the press conference held to announce the presentation of the Government's Human Fertilization and Embryology Bill, Mr Clarke said that his own conscience would require him to vote for embryo research. The Prime Minister, in a press interview, said that, in her view, Members of Parliament had a duty 'to take the very best scientific advice'.[79]

Under normal circumstances, the Government's Bill would have been considered first in the House of Commons and then passed to the Upper House. In this instance, the Government decided that the Bill's parliamentary passage would begin in the Lords. *New Scientist* reported, several months after the event, that the supporters of embryo research 'had helped to persuade the Government that the choice between the two clauses should be debated first in the calmer environment of the House of Lords'.[80] In another article, it was stated that those in favour of embryo research believed that this procedure 'could help defuse public emotions on the topic before the Bill is passed for discussion to the House of Commons'.[81] We have seen above that the pro-research lobby was more confident of receiving substantial support for embryo research in the Lords than in the Commons. Its success in persuading the Government to change the customary sequence was, therefore, a significant tactical achievement. For, in the first place, a clear victory for embryo research in the Lords might influence some of those in the Commons who were still undecided. Secondly, if the House of Lords were to endorse the clause permitting embryo research, this could be reversed in the Commons only by the addition of a new amendment, which would have to go back to the Upper House for approval.[82]

As the final stage in the struggle over embryo research got under way, the lobbying from both sides became increasingly intense. A pro-life conference was held to stimulate renewed activity. MPs were inundated with letters from members of LIFE and the SPUC 'asking us if we are going to allow ourselves to be murderers or not'.[83] At the same time, it was suggested that an amendment should be added to the Human Fertilization and Embryology Bill dealing with reform of the law on abortion.[84] Progress tried to counter these measures by arranging for Members of the House of Lords to be visited by families affected by genetic disease.[85] Announcements were made by the Medical Research Council and the British Medical Association reaffirming their support for embryo research.

In addition, the Royal Society took the unprecedented step of producing a 'fact sheet' about embryo research and of sending representatives to Westminster to explain informally to their Lordships why research involving human embryos should be allowed to continue.

In the first session in the Lords, on 7 December 1989, numerous eminent scientists appeared, for the first time in the long series of debates, to add their weight to the arguments in favour of research. The Archbishop of York, speaking personally, agreed with them that research on the pre-fourteen-day human embryo was defensible both biologically and morally.[86] No vote was taken after this debate. However, whilst thirty-four Members spoke in favour of embryo research, only twelve spoke against.[87] The impact of pro-research lobbying concerning the potential benefits of embryo research on the balance of opinion in the Lords was noted by Lord Prys-Davies:

There are some facts which I believe to be helpful and relevant. In my submission, those facts cannot be disregarded. They have been spelt out in letters from the Royal Society, from the MRC, the genetic group, and they are set out in the useful booklet issued last month by the Interim Licensing Authority . . . We are reminded there of the losses which will flow in the six main areas if a blanket prohibition is imposed upon embryo research. They have been referred to by so many people in the course of the debate that I need hardly spell them out again . . . Given the very great benefits that will flow from continued but carefully controlled research, on what grounds can one possibly justify the total banning of research?[88]

At its next meeting to discuss this topic, in February 1990, the Upper House approved, by 234 votes to 80, the clause allowing embryo research to continue under licence from a statutory body.

The jubilation of the supporters of embryo research over the vote in the Lords was tempered by uncertainty about what might happen in the Commons.[89] The members of the anti-research lobby also looked ahead, in their case defiantly, to the next step in the parliamentary process. The SPUC declared that the result in the Lords was a disappointment, but not a surprise. 'I think we will win when MPs vote on it in the House of Commons,' its spokesman said. 'The majority of MPs are sufficiently independently minded not to feel that the vote in the Lords demands their subservience.'[90] The political columnist of *New Scientist* judged the mood of the Commons to be more favourable to embryo research. He reported that his earlier gloom concerning the probable outcome of debate on this topic in the Commons was, at last, beginning to dissipate.[91] However, when the first debate in the Commons took place, on 2 April 1990, the result was inconclusive. For the thirteen speakers who supported embryo research on this occasion were matched by twelve who rejected such research. Unlike the Lords, where the first debate had shown clearly that the House was in favour of embryo research, the Commons seemed to be fairly evenly divided. With three weeks to go before the decisive parliamentary session, neither MPs nor outside observers could tell which way the Lower House would vote.[92]

At this late stage, the Human Fertilization and Embryology Bill was amended by the addition of a clause on abortion. This clause, which proposed that the upper time-limit for legal abortion be reduced from twenty-eight weeks to twenty-four weeks, was introduced on behalf of the Government by the Deputy Prime Minister. Other MPs then tabled further amendments which proposed even lower limits. These amendments were scheduled for discussion on the day after that set aside for consideration of the alternative clauses on embryo research.[93] Many of those in favour of embryo research were disturbed by this enlargement of the scope of the Bill. *Nature* reported that pro-research groups were afraid that the strong emotions associated with the long-standing abortion debate would spill over into discussion of embryo research and cloud the issues.[94] In *Nature*'s editorial column, it was acknowledged that there was a powerful case for reducing the time-limit for abortion.[95] But the editor described the inclusion of a clause on abortion in this particular Bill as 'both deplorable and mystifying'. He went on to wonder why the Government had chosen to 'complicate and perhaps even jeopardize the passage of its own legislation by converting that into a Trojan horse for the carriage of an amendment of abortion law'.[96]

This question cannot be answered with any confidence, although there are indications that the anti-abortion lobby had agreed to reciprocate by withholding further legislative proposals on abortion for some time to come.[97] It is clear, however, that, as a consequence of the introduction of the new clause, the pro-life lobby came to be as much concerned with its traditional topic of abortion as with embryo research during the last, critical, weeks before the Commons debate. For many of those opposed to research on human embryos, the two topics could not be separated and it was assumed that tactics that encouraged opposition to abortion would also serve to foster opposition to embryo research. As a result, the parliamentary campaign organized by the anti-abortion lobby culminated in the distribution to all MPs, on the day of the debate over embryo research, which was also the day before the debate over abortion, of a life-sized model of a twenty-week-old fetus. It seems that many MPs found this action distasteful. It is possible that its major effect was to make certain 'wavering' MPs react by voting in favour of embryo research.[98]

The pro-research lobby was not distracted by the topic of abortion, but concentrated exclusively upon embryo research. Progress tried to make sure that every MP was visited before the final debate either by an infertile couple or by someone who suffered from congenital abnormality.[99] The Genetic Interest Group, in co-ordination with Progress, focused its attention during the closing weeks on seventy-five MPs who seemed still to be undecided and open to persuasion.[100] It was generally agreed that the most effective tactic was to continue to explain to MPs what medical benefits would ensue if embryo research were to be allowed to continue.[101] This message was strengthened dramatically in the week before the Commons vote when Professor Robert Winston, head of the Hammersmith Infertility Clinic and also president of Progress, chose to announce that his group had developed techniques that made it possible to begin to screen IVF embryos for sex-linked genetic diseases. Just five days before the Commons vote, Professor Winston's picture appeared in the national press alongside the pregnant women who would be the first to benefit from these techniques when they gave birth to healthy children in four months' time. MPs were reminded of this exciting therapeutic advance and media coup in the course of the Commons debate.

Three women carriers of severe genetic disorders have been in the news recently. They are proud and happy because research has meant that they can have a baby free from handicap . . . Two of those families already have handicapped sons whom they love very dearly, as we saw in the press. However, they are now delighted to learn that they will be able to have girls who will be free of the genetic disorder that affects boys . . . If our crucial vote tonight had taken place last year and research had been banned, those happy mothers and their husbands would have been denied that chance. So much again for the so-called pro-life stance. It is restrictive and, I believe, the antithesis to life.[102]

At the end of the debate, the House of Commons approved the clause permitting the continuation of embryo research by 364 votes to 193. Both sides were surprised that the majority in favour of research in the Commons was so large. Some participants suggested that many of the uncommitted had been alienated by the heated and confusing rhetoric of the anti-research lobby. Others emphasized the efficiency of the campaign in support of embryo research.[103] The MP Tam Dalyell explained the pro-research victory in terms of a combination of political factors. In the first place, he wrote, the lobbying for embryo research was well organized and sustained. Secondly, the transfer of the opening debates, and the first vote, from the Commons to the Lords was, in his view, of considerable importance. The debate in the Upper House, he observed, 'created a different atmosphere from the ethos it would have had, had it come to the Commons first'.[104] Thirdly, Dalyell argued, embryo research was supported by a number of influential and persuasive politicians. In particular, he gave credit to Mr Clarke, the Secretary of State for Health, who introduced the Bill in the Commons; and to Mrs Thatcher who, although she did not speak, made 'it clear from an early stage that she would vote in favour of research'.[105]

Professor Winston preferred, in his celebratory reflections, to focus less on parliamentary tactics than on the actual achievements of those involved in embryo research. He suggested that there had been a significant shift in parliamentary opinion during the final week. This had occurred, in his judgment, as a direct result of the announcement of the first successful screening for sex-linked genetic diseases. The balance of parliamentary opinion had been decisively altered, he maintained, by this clear demonstration that research on human embryos really does produce genuine therapeutic benefits.[106]

3

Political parties and ministerial tactics

In the opening debates following the Warnock Report in 1984, the organized movement opposed to embryo research pressed the Government to introduce appropriate legislation without delay. Government speakers in both Houses accepted that legislation on embryo research was urgently needed and promised that legislative action would be taken soon.[1] In subsequent parliamentary sessions, Government representatives were regularly required to explain why this promise had not been kept. It was suggested that the Government had adopted a policy of 'making consultation a substitute for action'[2] with the aim of frustrating the wishes of the parliamentary majority.

The Government's reply to such criticism was, firstly, that they were internally divided and held no position in common which could provide the basis for legislation on embryo research.[3] Secondly, Government speakers insisted that, even if they had been able to agree among themselves, they would still have been unable to act quickly because of the absence of agreement among other parliamentarians.[4] Government representatives maintained that the Government were obliged to remain neutral with respect to an issue that cut across conventional party lines and about which there was no settled view. They argued that they had no real alternative but to promote further debate and to await patiently, along with other Members, the eventual resolution of initial differences of opinion.[5]

The two central themes in the Government's defence of their own actions were 'neutrality' and 'consensus'. The latter was the more fundamental in the sense that it was said to be the lack of agreement that obliged the Government to remain neutral and to delay legislation. The ultimate justification for the extended parliamentary process was that it would enable the Government, in due course, to enact legislation that would give expression to an unforced parliamentary consensus.[6]

It is doubtful, however, whether there was greater parliamentary consensus in 1989, when the Government finally acted, than in 1985 or 1986, when they refused to do so. It is possible that the level of agreement was less at the end of the lengthy sequence of appraisal than at the beginning. For example, the Commons vote against embryo research in 1985 was carried by a ratio of four to one, compared to the modest two-to-one majority for research achieved in the final Commons debate. It is true that the number of MPs who voted was much smaller in 1985 than in 1990.[7] But low attendance is characteristic of Private Member's Bills for procedural reasons; and Powell's Bill received much more support than is usual for Bills of this kind.[8] Although it is clear that parliamentary opinion moved significantly in favour of embryo research between 1984 and 1990, this change in the balance of opinion was not accompanied by an increase in the level of parliamentary consensus. Parliament seems to have remained just as deeply divided on this issue, but upon different lines. On several occasions, Government speakers admitted that they did not expect Parliament to reach an agreement about embryo research.[9] It is not surprising, therefore, that the eventual Government Bill included alternative clauses on such research, in order to cater for opposing views. The use of this device shows that the legislation introduced by the Government on this topic was not intended to be an expression of parliamentary consensus, but rather of whichever assessment of embryo research was dominant when the Bill was enacted.

The fact that legislation was introduced at a time when marked differences persisted concerning embryo research demonstrates that parliamentary unanimity was not a prerequisite for legislative action by the Government. This leads us to ask why the Government were unwilling to legislate during the early years when there was a substantial parliamentary majority that rejected embryo research. Why was it impossible to fulfil the promise of quick legislation by presenting to Parliament in, say 1986 rather than 1989, a Government Bill including the two alternative clauses on embryo research that were eventually used to enable parliamentarians to express their conflicting opinions on this difficult issue?

Ministerial tactics

Part of the answer, I suggest, is that some of those responsible for Government policy on this matter regarded the views of the early majority against embryo research as an unsuitable basis for legislation. As a result, they prolonged the process of consultation and debate in order to allow time for this mistaken majority to be replaced by what the Minister for

Health in 1985 called a 'right-minded majority', that is, a majority in favour of embryo research.

This interpretation implies that certain influential figures acting for Government were not, in practice, neutral with respect to the legislative outcome on embryo research. At a personal level, this is undeniable and was acknowledged by various speakers during the debates. For example, the Secretary of State for Health stated in the course of the Second Reading of the Government's Bill: 'I have never made any secret of the fact that I am an enthusiastic supporter of embryo research and, by coincidence, so is my hon. Friend the Minister for Health.'[10] In fact, all four MPs who spoke for the Government on this issue in the Commons voted in favour of embryo research in 1990. In the Lords, two of the three Government speakers who voted in 1990 also supported embryo research.

Government representatives maintained, however, that a distinction could be drawn between their personal convictions and the position adopted by the Government. They insisted that when they spoke on behalf of Government and when they made administrative decisions regarding the conduct of the debate – for instance, whether or not it was time to place legislation before Parliament – they remained completely detached and impartial.[11] These claims, I suggest, are undermined by the evidence contained in the parliamentary record. The evidence shows that Government representatives, despite their assertions of official neutrality, frequently spoke in the public setting of parliamentary debate in ways that tended to strengthen the position of embryo research. It is difficult not to infer that their belief in the legitimacy of such research must also have influenced those crucial decisions concerning Government strategy with respect to the embryo debate that were removed from critical public scrutiny.

Evidence of Government speakers' inclination towards embryo research occurs repeatedly in the debates in both Houses. In the first place, there was a tendency for such speakers to defend embryo research when it was under attack. For instance, in the opening debate in the Lords, eighteen of the non-Government speakers denounced experimentation on human embryos and only four spoke in its favour. When Lord Glenarthur rose to sum up the debate, however, although he noted the widespread abhorrence aroused in the House by the idea of such research, he chose, on behalf of the Government, to 'put the other side of the picture and say a little about the case for research'.[12] Similarly protective reactions can be found in Government speakers' contributions to the Commons debate on the Warnock Report and to the debate over the Bill presented by Mr Powell.[13] These interventions in support of embryo research might be regarded, in isolation, as illustrations of Government speakers seeking impartially to redress the balance of parliamentary discussions which had become too one-sided. But this interpretation is made untenable by the fact that Government speakers never argued against embryo research when the supporters of such research outnumbered its critics. Government representatives sought to maintain parliamentary balance only when those favouring embryo research appeared to be losing the argument.

In addition to this evidence of partiality, it is clear that Government officials often failed to maintain an even balance between the two sides when they delivered the opening speeches at major parliamentary sessions. In December 1989, for instance, Lord Mackay, the Lord Chancellor, initiated the parliamentary examination of the Government's Human Fertilization and Embryology Bill. He noted that 'it is not part of my function as a spokesman for the Government to make any judgment about the balance' of argument for and against embryo research.[14] Nevertheless, although his Lordship made no such judgment explicitly, he did pay much more attention to those arguments that supported embryo research, devoting exactly twice as many column-inches to exposition of the case for embryo research as he did to exposition of the case against. The Lord Chancellor was aware of this imbalance, but dismissed it as unimportant on the grounds that 'length of argument does not necessarily win over succinctness'.[15]

A similar situation can be observed in the final Commons debate in which the Secretary of State for Health spent more than twice as much time explaining the reasons for supporting embryo research as he did outlining the reasons given for opposing such research. Once again, the Government speaker offered an unconvincing apology for this obvious lack of even-handedness: 'I shall now, in fairness, remind the House of the arguments against embryo research – although I shall do so briefly, as others, inspired by deep convictions, will put the arguments more eloquently than I can.'[16] This self-justification is weak because speakers on *both* sides were presumably able to present their own cases with eloquence and deep conviction. It was, therefore, the task of the neutral Government representative to introduce the debate in a balanced manner with equal care given to the two opposing sets of considerations, rather than to leave those with whom the Minister happened to disagree to fend largely for themselves.

Government speakers tried to maintain the formal distinction between detached ministerial exposition and committed personal judgment. But this distinction tended to evaporate in practice as speakers' personal opinions became inextricably entangled with official accounts of the conflicting perspectives on embryo research.[17] As a result of this confusion, the very purpose of the parliamentary debate came to be officially defined in a manner that presupposed that research on human embryos should be allowed to continue. For example, Norman Fowler, the Secretary of State for Health in 1984, described the main objective of the parliamentary process as the provision of a 'satisfactory framework within which we can release the benefits of medical advance'.[18] In 1988 Tony Newton, the Minister for Health, depicted the parliamentary debate in a similar fashion as directed towards the production of 'a framework which will allow the proper use of the knowledge that we have, or can gain, to assist people to a sense of fulfilment in their lives, while clearly protecting the fundamental values on which our society is based'.[19]

These formulations assume, in their references to 'releasing the benefits of medical advance' and 'allowing the use of knowledge that we can gain', that Parliament must eventually permit scientists to engage in embryo research for therapeutic ends. This assumption was at the heart of almost all Government speeches.[20] Such a conception of the ultimate purpose of the debate was not neutral. It was fundamentally opposed to the position adopted by the many critics of embryo research, who argued that its possible benefits would simply have to be forgone because research of this kind could not be reconciled with the fundamental values on which our society is based, and who consequently argued that the legislative outcome of the parliamentary process should be the complete prohibition of this line of scientific inquiry.[21]

For Government speakers, committed by their understanding of the purpose of the debate to the eventual release of scientific benefits, the opposition movement could not be regarded as a proper consensus on which to base legislation, even though it might have majority support, but only as an ill-considered and passing reaction.

The achievement of the Warnock committee was that it was able, even with its diverse views, to put together laboriously a report which could be put to the public. Inevitably, this House has gone in the opposite direction. In the debate, most hon. Members have shown strong feelings of considerable depth and tended to advocate their own feelings. In a sense, they have taken apart the agreement reached in the report. Indeed, many hon. Members have denounced the conclusions of the report. As we take the matter further, we shall have to strive to get nearer to some consensus.[22]

Within a few moments of uttering these words Mr Clarke, then Minister for Health and subsequently Secretary of State for Health, replaced 'getting nearer some consensus' with the aim of establishing a 'right-minded majority'. By 'right-minded', he clearly meant a majority that agreed with him and his close colleagues that experiments involving human embryos should, in due course, be given a legal charter. The long series of consultations and debates that followed these early confrontations, for which Mr Clarke was directly responsible,[23] was made to continue until his 'right-minded majority' had been given time to form.[24]

The first debates in which the majority of speakers spoke in favour of embryo research occurred early in 1988. At the end of the debate in January of that year, we find Lord Skelmersdale concluding in the Upper House that 'your Lordships have pretty well decided the issue [of embryo research] today. The tally is that four out of the 21 speakers have come down firmly against research in any form of the word, whereas the rest are prepared to accept it.'[25] At this juncture, it seemed to those responsible for Government policy that the time for legislative action was finally drawing near. Lord Skelmersdale clearly drew this inference from the favourable discussion in the Lords: 'I thought that there was a strong feeling emerging from today's debate that, while there is still plenty of scope for debating the detail . . . all are agreed that there must be some kind of legislation soon . . . we intend to legislate in this Parliament.'[26] Given the apparent change in the balance of parliamentary opinion, it was no longer unrealistic to envisage that legislation might be passed that would make embryo research legitimate and secure the release of its potential benefits. In these altered circumstances, the Government's promise to legislate within the current Parliament was fulfilled.

Divisions within the party of government

The parliamentary representatives of the Conservative Party were, on the whole, opposed to embryo research. In 1985, 48 per cent of Conservative MPs went into the division lobbies after the debate on the Powell Bill. Of these Members, 89 per cent voted against further research on human IVF embryos. In 1986, 57 per cent of Conservative MPs voted on this topic and 83 per cent of them cast their vote in favour of the immediate prohibition of such research.[27] There was, however, an influential minority within the Conservative Party that was unwilling to endorse this wholly negative reaction to embryo research. This minority view, as we have seen, was prevalent among the Conservative ministers directly responsible for legislation on embryo research, and it was this view that was eventually put into effect in the Human Fertilization and Embryology Act.

These contrasting responses to embryo research within the Conservative Party can be traced to differences of political viewpoint which have existed for many years. Normally, in relation to issues that are covered by the official agenda of the party, the impact of these internal divisions is kept to a minimum by means of the established procedures for maintaining party discipline.[28] However, when important questions of conscience come before

Parliament, there is a convention that disciplinary restraints should be lifted and that MPs should be free to vote according to their personal preference, even when the issues arise from Government legislation.[29] This convention was adopted by the Government in relation to embryo research, despite demands from many Conservative backbenchers that their rejection of such research should become the official policy of the party. Consequently, in the absence of a clear party line and with disciplinary mechanisms in abeyance, the Conservative Party became openly divided on this issue in accordance with certain fundamental differences of political perspective which exist among its members.[30]

It is possible to identify numerous ideological sub-groupings within the modern Conservative Party.[31] But the issue of embryo research necessarily separated those Conservatives who took an active interest in this topic into two broad categories, namely, those who were inclined to vote for the continuation of embryo research and those who preferred to vote against. The views expressed by these two groupings correspond closely to the division between 'traditional Conservatism' and 'progressive Conservatism' which is common to all typologies dealing with Conservative ideology and internal differentiation.

Conservative thought has always been centrally concerned with the balance between continuity and change that may be achieved by means of political action.[32] Traditional Conservatism emphasizes the need for continuity of social life and the maintenance of established values. It is from this commitment to stability and order that the political use of the term 'conservative' derives. The basic features of the traditional Conservative position have been summarized as follows:

An undeniable characteristic of the Conservative disposition is a reluctance to change what is known for what is assumed or claimed to be better. For the future is unknowable and the human is not such an omniscient being that he can account for all the factors involved in any extreme surgery of present structures . . . The purpose of political change . . . is to conserve the rights and liberties of an actual society, to maintain those institutions which embody those rights and liberties . . . [Conservatism] agonizes about change and is sceptical about its beneficial consequences.[33]

Following from these assumptions and concerns, the traditional Conservative preference is for small-scale, manageable change which brings modest improvements to people's lives without involving major alteration to the existing social order. Many Conservatives were deeply disturbed, therefore, by the sudden arrival of powerful techniques which made possible the widespread redistribution of living human organisms outside the womb and which led to the proposal that some of these embryonic human entities be made available for purposes of experimentation. Embryo research and assisted reproduction were seen as radical departures from established practice which contravened fundamental human rights; which threatened the long-standing structure of family life on which orderly social existence depends; and which could easily lead towards a world in which the collective wisdom embodied in existing institutions would be over-turned, with disastrous results, as science intervened increasingly in human affairs. The dynamic of social change was seen as being in danger of accel-erating out of control as science began to focus its amoral gaze upon the most intimate and morally sensitive areas of human conduct. Many Conservative MPs looked into a possible future in which embryo research had been given free reign, and recoiled in horror.

The scientific world has come a long way in the past two or three years from the first-test tube baby, to womb leasing and to the possibility of baby manufacturing. I and many other people find it incredibly frightening that the moral, legal and social aspects of these developments remain largely unrecognized, little considered and unable to adapt to scientific progress. If the Government do not act now – this year, this month or even this week – we shall merely encourage exploitation, mis-management and social disaster . . . If we allow multiple fertilization, do we allow the doctors to discard unwanted or imperfect human embryos? Do we allow embryos to be grown merely for research? Will we in the future allow the growth of human embryos in laboratories for use as spare part supplies of tissues and organs? . . . Will society accept the sale and purchase of human embryos – an embryo mar-keting board? The ideas are horrific.[34]

A large proportion of Conservatives in Parliament responded anxiously to these actual and possible developments, in accordance with the traditional Conservative ethos. They insisted that society would be unable to cope unless the process was scaled down, brought under parliamentary control and made compatible with existing beliefs and values. Embryo research was singled out as a subject of special concern by most Conservative speakers, partly because its apparent disregard for the humanity of IVF embryos was seen as a fundamental violation of the established moral order, but also because it was identified as the moving force that would be ultimately responsible for the social and moral problems that lay ahead. Most Conservative MPs were willing to allow the continued use of IVF for the benefit of infertile couples – as long as this was done within what they regarded as the normal setting of the heterosexual family.[35] But it was widely believed within the party that drastic action was needed in order to prevent embryo research from producing a cumulative sequence of further innovations which would erode values and social practices that were essen-tial to any civilized society.

Although traditional Conservatism has always provided the central strand in Conservative ideology, there has also been a movement within the party, at least since the Second World War, that can be called 'progressive Conservatism'.[36] Those involved in this movement have sought to adapt Conservative principles to the modern world, instead of attempting to resist the advance of the modern world in defence of Conservative principles.[37] There has been some antagonism between traditional and progressive Conservatives. The progressive wing has sometimes been denounced as 'but a milder shade of the collectivist, reformist philosophy of the Socialist establishment'.[38] Nevertheless, progressive Conservatives have been influential within the modern party and have striven to encourage the formation of policies that channel the main currents of social development in a Conservative direction, that is, along a judicious middle way between the ideological extremes of British political life.[39]

The reformist perspective of the progressive Conservatives is well exemplified in the views of Government speakers and other Conservative MPs in favour of embryo research. This minority regarded the unease of most of their colleagues as quite unjustified and as arising from an unthinking commitment to the status quo. The progressives were confident that the potential benefits of embryo research could be enjoyed without unleashing irreversible processes of social disruption. They tended to assume that all rational, right-minded people would come to see this in due course. They firmly rejected the view adopted by the Conservative majority that the continuation of research on human embryos would place society on a slippery slope towards moral bankruptcy. Nevertheless, they tried to reassure their parliamentary colleagues by emphasizing that they would support embryo research only if it was to be carried out with 'proper controls and with good purposes'.[40]

The progressives argued that 'as long as embryo research is done openly and within a framework of strict statutory controls . . . the benefits that are held in promise by that research should not be witheld from those who wish to take advantage of them'.[41] They stressed that, in supporting such research, they sought to contribute to social progress by advancing the cause of rational, scientific thought. At the same time, they insisted, they were determined to channel and to regulate these developments in such a way that the products of embryo research would be used to strengthen the role of the traditional family and to maintain what they saw as the values of a humane society.[42]

This moderately progressive reasoning provided the rationale for the strategy adopted by Government ministers of delaying the legislative process in order to make time for the emergence of a more considered and, hence, more sympathetic assessment of embryo research. It was also characteristic of that small group of twenty-two Conservatives that voted against Mr Powell's Bill in 1985.

I believe, as does my right hon. and learned Friend the Minister [Kenneth Clarke], that the evidence favours voting against Second Reading [Hon. Members: 'No'.] We must understand the advantages that will flow from continued experimentation, because unless we understand them we cannot form the moral judgments that are required. My right hon. and learned Friend identified them in broad terms: progress in the treatment of infertility; progress in the treatment of miscarriage; greater understanding of genetic disorders; and advancement in methods of contraception . . . Against that one must set the moral outrage that many people feel, and on this issue there are two important points to bear in mind. First, those of us who argue against the Bill . . . have never asked for and we do not want unlicensed or unsupervised experimentation. Secondly, I support the remarks of my right hon. and learned Friend the Minister about the nature of the being with which we are dealing. I must tell [Mr Powell] that to call this the Unborn Children (Protection) Bill is misleading.[43]

The reactions to embryo research within the Conservative Party were built around the two contrasting ideological positions outlined above. From the perspective of traditional Conservatism, research of this kind was an alien development which threatened to undermine cherished values and which had to be stopped before it was too late. From the perspective of progressive Conservatism, embryo research was a welcome product of the advance of rational thought which, once it was properly regulated, would lead to improvements in social life through the controlled production and release of therapeutic benefits.

The progressive response was dominant at the highest level of government. Not only did the ministers most centrally involved declare their progressive views early on, but the Prime Minister also made it clear that she was in favour of legislation based directly on the Warnock recommendations permitting licensed research.[44] In 1985, almost all members of Cabinet pointedly withheld their support from the anti-research legislation introduced by Mr Powell[45] in accordance with the view expressed by the Minister for Health that the Bill was precipitate and extreme.[46] In 1990, only four members of Cabinet voted against embryo research, whilst fourteen members voted for its continuation. Thus, throughout the period of parliamentary debate, there was significantly more support for embryo research within the Conservative Government than among Conservative parliamentarians as a whole.

Because many leading members of the Government were inclined towards embryo research, the negative reaction associated with the traditional Conservative viewpoint could not become the basis for Government policy. At the same time, the lack of support for such research among ordinary Conservatives meant that it was equally impossible for the progressives to implement the alternative policy of making embryo research legitimate. As a result of this political stalemate, the most that Government ministers could do was to delay the parliamentary process, to try to make sure that the case for embryo research was well publicized, to allow a free vote and to hope that 'right-minded thinking' would come to predominate, not only among Conservatives, but also among those from other political parties. In the absence of a firm legislative commitment by the Government, the fate of embryo research came to depend on the overall balance of parliamentary opinion and, in particular, on the degree of support for such research within the Labour Party.

Reactions to embryo research within the Labour Party

The Labour Party was by far the largest non-government party during the period under study. In 1985, the Conservatives had 397 seats in the House of Commons and the Labour Party 209. By 1990, the number of Labour MPs had increased by twenty.[47] The political ideology of the Labour Party is more forward looking than that of traditional Conservatism. Like other socialist parties, the British Labour Party is guided by the idea that the present pattern of social relationships can be transformed for the general good by means of political action. This is made clear in the party's constitution, which states that the focal aim of the Labour Party is 'to promote the political, social and economic emancipation of the people'.[48] Whereas Conservatism is said to appeal to a widespread distrust of the unknown,[49] the Labour Party is often claimed to be the party of the future. The Labour Party, however, is a party of moderate policies whose members have generally sought to bring about social progress by acting within the constraints of the existing parliamentary system.[50]

In the early debates on the Warnock Report and on the Unborn Children (Protection) Bill, most of the support for embryo research came from members of the Labour Party. These Labour speakers argued, like the progressive Conservatives, that fears about future misuse of science in this area were excessive and uninformed; that embryo research, if it were allowed to continue, would generate significant therapeutic benefits; and that these benefits would enhance the quality of domestic life for the population at large.

The criterion forming my view about the deliberations of the Warnock Report is that of the greater good that its recommendations afford our society. I will have no part in any lobby or argument whose recommendations will in practice discriminate, punish or prolong the needless misery of childlessness . . . Research into the following areas offers infertile women better diagnosis and treatment. The first aspect is spontaneous abortion . . . Research is needed to establish the precise conditions to maximize the chances of viability through full-time pregnancy. Success would mean less emotional trauma for the would-be mother and a reduction in needless medical expense and time in post- abortion care. Secondly, early detection of embryo abnormality and methods to perfect pre-implantation screening of *in vitro* embryos would reduce the unhappy consequences of the present system of late screening and subsequent abortion . . . Thirdly, research is needed into the origins and treatment of conditions that endanger the life of the newborn child . . . Much benefit will come to society with the reduction in the unhappiness associated with infertility. For those reasons, I believe that a limited and highly controlled amount of experimentation is permissible and beneficial to society.[51]

Progressive, utilitarian reasoning along these lines was used to justify immediate support for embryo research among a small number of Labour MPs. During the opening debates, however, the majority of socialists at Westminster, although not actively opposed to embryo research, displayed little interest in this topic or in the Warnock proposals generally.[52] When Powell's Bill came before the Commons several months later, only eighty-six Labour MPs voted, forty-four of whom agreed with the Conservative majority that further research on human embryos should be prohibited.[53] Thus, it quickly became clear that, not only was there widespread indifference, but there was also a significant body of principled resistance to embryo research within the Labour camp.[54]

In its initial reaction to embryo research, the parliamentary Labour Party divided into three distinct elements: a small group of ardent supporters; a similarly sized group of MPs strongly opposed to such research; and an inert majority whose political interests appeared to lie elsewhere. The Labour MPs in favour of embryo research were able to act with less restraint than the progressives within the Conservative Government. As a result, they were able to play a prominent part in sabotaging the Unborn Children (Protection) Bill during its final report stage.[55] Nevertheless, the existence of a number of Labour MPs who had voted for the Powell Bill seemed to suggest to certain Labour activists that the conservative reaction against the liberal reforms of preceding decades was no longer confined to parties of the right, but had begun to establish a foothold among the parliamentary representatives within their own party.[56] Consequently, at the next annual conference of the Labour Party, action was taken to condemn the offending MPs publicly and to try to bring them into line with the party's progressive ideology. This action took the form of a motion which was headed 'Reproductive rights', part of which is quoted below:

The Conference believes that the freedom to decide whether or not to bear children should be a woman's fundamental right . . . This Conference deplores the decision of 44 Labour Members of Parliament to vote for Enoch Powell's so-called 'Unborn Children (Protection) Bill' . . . This Conference is gravely concerned at the absence of party policy pertaining to women's reproductive rights, particularly since, during recent months, a number of new developments have occurred in the ongoing debate over a woman's right to control her reproductive power . . . Abandoning the idea that there can be 'conscience clauses' or free votes on such matters, the National Executive Committee should mount a concerted campaign.[57]

In the discussion that followed, it was argued that embryo research should be supported and encouraged because the techniques it would produce would confer on women greater control over their fertility. A second, subsidiary theme was that men within the Labour Party did not take 'women's issues' seriously and that this was the explanation for the low participation of Labour MPs in the parliamentary debates on Warnock and the Powell Bill:

I have come to the platform to say how amazed and disgusted I am at the number of men who could not wait to get out of this room as soon as this motion came to [be] debated . . . The priority that men have given within our party to the issues relating to women is a shame and a disgrace . . . when it comes to votes in Parliament the men in our party have to see this as a crucial issue and be there.[58]

The conference motion was carried by a large majority, but it did not commit the party to any specific action on embryo research.

In the Labour Party, unlike the Conservative Party, the opponents of embryo research were a beleaguered minority which could be denounced as ideologically deviant and as out of step with party policy on related issues, such as abortion and women's rights. The session at the annual conference in 1985 illustrates how ideological pressure of this kind was quickly brought to bear upon the small group of 'moral conservatives' within the party. This pressure may have had some effect on the subsequent pattern of voting on embryo research. For, when the Unborn Children (Protection) Bill reappeared in the Commons in October 1986, the number of Labour MPs voting against research fell from forty-four to thirty-one – even though there had been a 10 per cent increase in Labour participation. On the other hand, only one Labour MP actually changed from voting against to voting for embryo research during this period. Furthermore, half the Labour MPs in the Commons still took no part in the vote.[59] Thus, there was no sign of that great surge in active parliamentary support that had been called for at the conference. It appears that the demand for ideological conformity that occurred within the more reformist of the two main parties did not initiate the process of mass conversion that was required if embryo research was to become formally established in law.

This modest reaction to internal ideological pressure suggests that the substantial shift towards active support for embryo research that did eventually occur among Labour MPs was primarily due to outside influences. The fact that both political parties moved in the same direction, despite their marked differences in ideological configuration and internal dynamics, also suggests that the main factors producing these changes originated externally. Although the Labour Party and the Conservative Party differed considerably in their receptivity to the case for embryo research, the swing in favour of such research was very large in both instances. Between 1985 and 1990, the Conservatives moved from a situation in which 89 per cent of those who voted were against embryo research to one in which 57 per cent of voters supported its continuation. Over the same period, the Labour Party moved from having 51 per cent of its voters opposed to embryo research to a situation in which 84 per cent were in favour. Among MPs of all parties, 23.5 per cent of those who voted *against* embryo research in 1985 voted *for* such research in 1990. There was no movement at all in the other direction. In order to understand this significant increase in support for embryo research across the whole political spectrum, we must look more closely at the organized lobbying on behalf of research on human embryos which gathered momentum as the parliamentary debate proceeded.

4

The impact of the pro-research lobby

In the early debates that followed the presentation of the Warnock Report, the anti-abortion lobby encouraged and prepared speakers in both Houses to condemn embryo research and to demand legislation that would bring such research to an end. This active lobbying had a particularly powerful effect upon the numerically superior and ideologically receptive Conservative Party. As a result, the long-standing repertoire of anti-abortion arguments concerning the rights of the unborn and the importance of maintaining the traditional family was adopted by a large number of parliamentarians and reapplied to the new topic of research on human IVF embryos. In this way, the parliamentary debate over embryo research began as a virtual replay of prior debates over abortion reform. This time, however, the anti-abortionists/anti-embryo researchers were well organized and politically ascendant, whilst those in favour of research were unorganized, poorly prepared and in a parliamentary minority.

The anti-abortion lobby, like the ALRA two decades earlier, tried to take advantage of its parliamentary dominance by introducing a Private Member's Bill. But, unlike the ALRA, the anti-abortion lobby was confronted in Parliament by an experienced band of tactically skilled opponents. In addition, again unlike the ALRA, it had to deal with an unsympathetic Government whose officials repeatedly deferred the final decision about the fate of embryo research. In the 1960s, the anti-abortionists had suffered from the speed at which the Bill on abortion passed through Parliament. In the 1980s, they suffered from the prolonged legislative delay which gave their adversaries a full five years in which to organize, to develop and publicize their case, and to bring about a dramatic parliamentary reversal.

This delay enabled the pro-researchers eventually to win a clear parliamentary victory. But, at the outset, the scientific and medical establishment was unprepared for the battle to come. Its members were surprised and shocked by the bitter rejection of what *they* saw as Warnock's unduly cautious proposals for a restricted form of externally licensed embryo research.[1] Scientists only gradually came to realize that they would have to fight hard if research on human embryos was to survive at all. The organized campaign on behalf of embryo research, therefore, was slow to take shape, and it was not until the display of widespread parliamentary support for the Powell Bill that the need for positive action was finally recognized.

The first major step in the pro-research campaign was the formation in 1985 of the Voluntary Licensing Authority by the Medical Research Council and the Royal College of Obstetricians and Gynaecologists. This body was set up to regulate both embryo research and associated clinical practice on a voluntary basis. Its political objective was, in the words of *New Scientist*, 'to allay public disquiet over research on embryos, especially in the wake of the bill by Enoch Powell [that] is currently racing through Parliament'.[2] The VLA was intended to counter the accusation repeatedly advanced by the critics of embryo research in the early stages of debate that it would be impossible to monitor such research and that experimentation on human embryos would inevitably accelerate out of control. Throughout the latter part of the debate the VLA, later renamed the Interim Licensing Authority (ILA), was regularly cited in Parliament as having clearly shown that, even without statutory regulation, embryo research could develop in a careful, controlled manner, with no danger of erratic movement down a slippery slope towards social disruption or moral decay.[3]

Shortly after the formation of the VLA, the second crucial step was taken in defence of embryo research, with the creation of Progress. This body was established in order to campaign actively in Parliament and in the media in support of 'controlled research into human reproduction'.[4] It grew out of the 'crisis team' that had been set up by a 'handful of MPs, Doctors and individuals' to prevent the passage of the Powell Bill.[5] The minutes of the first annual general meeting of Progress, in June 1986, provides a list of forty-five members, drawn from agencies such as the Birth Control Campaign, the Pregnancy Advisory Service, the Christian Socialist Movement, the Labour Abortion Rights Campaign and the National Deaf–Blind Rubella Association. There were also four leading medical researchers and four MPs. The main impetus for the Progress campaign came from the representatives of scientific and medical research. The political members supplied the links through which these scientists and their lay supporters were able to exert influence upon parliamentary affairs.

From 1985 onwards, Progress, the VLA and the MRC worked together to raise the level of direct and indirect contact between parliamentarians and the scientists engaged in embryo research and in associated clinical practice. Members from both Houses were repeatedly invited to undertake visits of inspection to suitable clinics and research centres; and scientists and doctors made regular trips to Westminster to explain their case to the parliamentary decision-makers. Contact of this kind was supplemented by the systematic distribution of pro-research documents, by sustained epistolary pressure, by the organization of deputations to Government ministers, by the formation of local groups, and by co-operation with other bodies sympathetic to embryo research.[6] Gradually, the lobby for embryo research recovered from a shaky start and began to have a discernible impact upon parliamentary opinion.

The changing pattern of parliamentary opinion

The long-term shift that took place in parliamentarians' views of embryo research can be seen with particular clarity in the testimony of those speakers who openly changed their minds, as the sequence of debates unfolded, about the use of human embryos for experimental purposes. I will use the speeches of Lady Saltoun, who altered her views on embryo research three times, to illustrate the changing pattern of parliamentary opinion.[7] In the debate in the Lords in 1984, in response to the Warnock Report, Lady Saltoun spoke strongly against allowing embryo research to continue under any circumstances. In the debate in 1988 on the Government's White Paper,[8] she urged others to join her in supporting research of this kind. One year later, in a debate over a version of Powell's anti-research Bill, her Ladyship 'ate her words' and opposed experimentation involving human embryos. However, in 1990, she finally voted in favour of such research under the conditions laid down in the Government's Bill. Lady Saltoun is, thus, an intriguing example of a parliamentarian who participated actively in the initial rejection of embryo research as well as in its eventual collective endorsement, and who seems to have been swept back and forth by the currents of opinion and social influence at work in the embryo debate.

In 1984, Lady Saltoun spoke as follows:

I come now to the vexed question of whether research on human embryos should be permitted at all or only up to a certain age. I do not know when the soul enters the body and I do not believe anyone else knows, either . . . Until we know beyond all shadow of doubt, I think that the answer must be no to all experimentation on human embryos . . . If we leave that door open any longer we shall never get it shut again . . . And then, sooner than we realise – because of the speed of scientific development – we shall have experiments in inter-species breeding and genetic engineering with a view to creating a master race . . . not to mention a growing disregard for the sanctity of human life. Tempting as it is to say the ills of this world are such that no path which could lead to the alleviation of some of them should remain untrodden, there must be some roads down which we do not go.[9]

The arguments against embryo research employed in this passage are typical of those that dominated the opening debates.[10] Lady Saltoun's most fundamental point is that it is difficult to deny the human embryo the spiritual, and hence the moral, status of a full human being. The implication, which she leaves unstated but which was made clear by numerous other speakers, is that this status carries with it the natural right not to be used as an experimental subject for others' benefit. Secondly, she emphasizes that the contravention of human rights involved in experimentation on embryos makes such research wrong in principle – no matter how much it might lead to 'alleviation of the ills of this world'. In other words, for Lady Saltoun, as for most speakers in the early debates, the essential humanity of the early embryo made it impossible to justify embryo research by reference to the medical advances that such research might generate.

In her metaphor of 'trying to shut the door' on embryo research, Lady Saltoun treats research of this kind as breaching an important moral boundary. Her view appears to be that, if this boundary is crossed, it will become increasingly difficult to prevent science from extending the scope of its activities in ways that will further undermine essential values. She mentions 'inter-species breeding and genetic engineering' as the kinds of activities she has in mind. Such practices were taken by her Ladyship, as well as by many other speakers, to illustrate the undeniably immoral developments that would follow in due course from the pursuit of embryo research.[11] Finally, it seems to be implied in these criticisms that the scientists involved in embryo research cannot be trusted to judge the moral character of their own conduct and that the ultimate decision about the legitimacy of embryo research should be made, not by these technical experts, but by lay persons whose moral and spiritual judgment will be undistorted by personal commitment to the scientific enterprise.

Lady Saltoun's initial arguments were characteristic of the early opposition to embryo research. The revisions she made in subsequent speeches show how the tenor of parliamentary debate began slowly to change as the actions of the pro-research lobby took effect. This is Lady Saltoun speaking in 1988:

I have taken steps to inform myself on the exact nature of the so-called embryo research which is being done. I have visited . . . Medical Research Council laboratories . . . where the research is done, the Infertility Clinic . . . in Edinburgh . . . and the Cromwell Hospital . . . where I saw the various processes involved in *in vitro* fertilization being carried out. I am most grateful to the directors and professors who made these visits possible . . . If the research now being carried out involved the murder of a child it could not be allowed under the law; but having seen what I have seen and learnt what I have learnt I do not believe that it does. In fact I am inclined to the view that up until the appearance of the primitive streak the pre-embryo cannot be regarded as a human being . . . Therefore, I feel extremely hesitant to ban, for no good reason, research which promises . . . to enable couples who are particularly at risk of having children with serious genetic abnormalities to have defective pre-embryos rejected, thereby reducing the number of handicapped children who are born.[12]

One critical difference between Lady Saltoun's speeches in 1984 and 1988 is that, by the later date, she had made direct contact with the experts whose activities she had previously condemned from a distance. In this respect, she was in no way unusual. Many parliamentarians visited clinics or research centres after the early debates and most of them, like Lady Saltoun, returned to Parliament to speak enthusiastically on behalf of embryo research. As Lady Saltoun's case illustrates, this enthusiasm was released by a significant redefinition of the human embryo. The basic source of Lady Saltoun's opposition to embryo research in her initial speech had been the notion that the early embryo was morally indistinguishable from more mature human beings. By 1988, however, what she had 'seen and learnt' among the scientists seems to have convinced her that the entity investigated in this line of research was not even a proper embryo, let alone an emergent human being with a soul. Thus Lady Saltoun, as a result of her contact with the scientific community, was led, like many others, to adopt the newly invented concept of the 'pre-embryo' and consequently to abandon her original conclusion that embryo research was wrong in principle.[13]

Acceptance of scientists' definition of the experimental subject of embryo research made such research permissible. It also made it possible for Lady Saltoun, and for others whose initial opposition had been weakened in this way, to take account of the benefits of such research. Lady Saltoun had previously dismissed the original practical aim of embryo research, that is, the provision of children for the infertile, as relatively trivial and, quite apart from the moral difficulties, as not worth the expenditure of taxpayers' money.[14] In her Ladyship's later speech, however, embryo research was seen to be justified, not by its contribution to the reduction of infertility, but by the promise of effective control over the transmission of genetic abnormalities.

Lady Saltoun seems to have changed sides in the debate because she had talked to the technical experts and because she had come to accept their estimate of the likely benefits of embryo research as well as their account of the nature of the early human embryo. As she put it in a later parliamentary session: 'I was fascinated and deeply impressed by the scientists I met [and] I found [their] arguments enormously persuasive.'[15] Despite this tribute to those engaged in embryo research, Lady Saltoun reverted in her next speech to her original position, on the grounds that the scientists' case, although highly plausible, had not been proven conclusively. There was, she said, still room for doubt about the true nature of the human embryo and, for this reason, the embryo must be protected.[16] Nevertheless, her Ladyship did eventually vote in favour of embryo research in 1990; unfortunately, without explaining to the House why she had changed her mind yet again. It is reasonable to presume, however, that her justifications for voting for research would have been similar to the views expressed in her pro-research speech of 1988. Indeed, these views were held essentially in common by the growing number of parliamentarians who spoke in support of embryo research during the later stages of debate.

It is evident from the parliamentary record that the pro-research lobby succeeded in bringing about a sharp increase in contact between parliamentary representatives and the scientists involved in embryo research. In the debates in 1985-6, there was no mention of contact of this kind. As the debates continued, increasing reference was made to consultations with scientists, to visits by scientists to Westminster, and to visits of inspection by Members of both Houses to IVF clinics and research units. During the critical debates in 1989-90, one in three of those who spoke for research mentioned, in the course of their addresses, that they had discussed these matters directly with members of the scientific community. In contrast, only one in twelve of those opposed to embryo research referred to personal contact of this kind.[17]

Throughout the parliamentary debate over embryo research, the arguments of those consistently opposed to such research remained essentially unchanged. The case developed by the pro-research lobby, however, altered significantly as the struggle continued, in that increasing emphasis was placed on the possibility of using techniques produced by means of embryo research to prevent the transmission of genetic disease. In the following passage from a Commons debate in 1990, a staunch supporter of embryo research and a member of Progress thanks 'scientists and doctors' for their help and then attempts to clarify how research on human embryos would be able to contribute to a major reduction in the frequency of inherited disability:

We are not scientists or doctors and must rely on informed opinions. I am grateful ... for the information that has landed in enormous quantities on our desks ... We are all better informed than we were even two weeks ago, and certainly more informed than we were one or two years ago. No right hon. or hon. Member could fail to be impressed by the representations made by the large number of genetic interest groups . . . I am grateful for the representations that I have received from people, including doctors and scientists, who know of my strong position in favour of embryo research . . . Let us be clear what pre-embryo research could achieve . . . The objective is to identify and offer help to people who are at risk of passing on a genetic disorder . . . by taking a single cell from the developing conceptus after fertilization *in vitro* before replacing the pre-embryo in the mother. Only pre-embryos which were free from genetic disease would be replaced so that the woman could start her pregnancy knowing that her baby would not be affected.[18]

We can see here how the case for embryo research came to focus, for long-standing advocates of such research as well as for more recent converts such as Lady Saltoun, upon the use of IVF techniques to eliminate defective embryos for couples who were known to be liable to transmit genetic abnormalities. This powerful justification for the continuation of embryo research, originating from within the scientific community, was a central theme in pro-research lobbying and became increasingly prominent during the later phases of the parliamentary process. For instance, as we saw in chapter 2, Progress brought its campaign to a climax by arranging for a visit to Westminster by 200 families affected by genetic disease and by announcing the imminent arrival of the first babies to benefit from selective IVF screening for sex-linked genetic defects.[19] As a result of such activities, in the crucial debates in late 1989 and early 1990, 75 per cent of those arguing for embryo research made significant reference to its potential contribution to the prevention of genetic disorder.

In the early debates, reference to control of genetic disease had been a minor feature of those few pro-research speeches in which it was mentioned, and had been used as a justification for embryo research only in general terms with no detailed account of how genetic control was to be achieved.[20] During later pro-research speeches, the use of IVF techniques to control the transmission of genetic disease was often the central topic, and the technical procedures to be employed in such control were repeatedly elaborated in detail. Many speakers devoted the greater part of their speeches to describing the horrors of congenital abnormality along with the enormous increase in human happiness that would follow from a reduction in its frequency. Many others, as in the example below, made it clear that acceptance of a direct link between embryo research and control over genetic disorder had been decisive in leading them to vote for research. None of the other possible benefits of embryo research were ever emphasized in this way.

My first reaction, believing as I do as a Christian in the sanctity of life was that there should be no research; it should be prohibited . . . However, after visiting one of the units engaged in this work, and seeing what is done . . . I am now convinced that research on embryos up to 14 days should be allowed, provided of course that it is strictly controlled . . . The principal reason for my view that embryo research should be allowed up to 14 days is that such research can make an important contribution to preventing the creation of grossly deformed and mentally handicapped babies.[21]

This kind of testimony had been entirely absent from the early debates in which embryo research had been overwhelmingly rejected. In the later debates, it was the dominant feature of the case successfully presented in Parliament on behalf of such research.

Genetic control and social control

The pro-research lobby succeeded in tipping the balance of parliamentary opinion in favour of embryo research during the later stages of debate by promising wide-ranging control over the transmission of human genes. In the early debates, in contrast, it had been the opponents of embryo research who had seized on the topic of genetic control and who had used the threat of genetic manipulation as a weapon with which to attack the Warnock recommendations in support of such research.[22]

Your Lordships have been speaking with great effect about experimenting with embryos. Can we not expect, perhaps, that this will lead to juggling with genes? Is it not possible that in time to come people may be able to order their own children? Someone may say, 'All right; I'll have two boys with blue eyes', or, 'I will have two girls with golden hair'. What a terrible thought![23]

The initial outcry against the dangers of genetic engineering was so vigorous and so widespread that it quickly came to be accepted that science could be permitted to proceed no further in this direction. This view was adopted, not only by those opposed to embryo research, but also by its supporters, who insisted that such research was not intended to lead, and would never be allowed to lead, to the active construction or redesign of human individuals.[24] As a result, when the Government's White Paper was published in 1987, it added several clauses explicitly forbidding research of this kind to the proposals contained in the Warnock Report.

One of the greatest causes of public disquiet has been the perceived possibility that newly developed techniques will allow the artificial creation of human beings with certain pre-determined characteristics through modification of an early embryo's genetic structure. The technical prospects for achieving this are in fact extremely remote, even if anyone wished to undertake such work. Nevertheless, it is a procedure which society would clearly regard as ethically unacceptable, and the Bill will prohibit it.[25]

By the end of the first phase of parliamentary debate, the prohibition of genetic engineering had become part of the moral framework within which embryo research was required to operate and within which justifications for such research had to be formulated. Thus, although the initial debates produced no agreement about the legitimacy of research on early human embryos, they did establish that if such research was to be justified to any degree by reference to techniques of genetic control, these techniques would have to stop short of direct genetic manipulation of human individuals.

This was the context in which, after the publication of the White Paper, the pro-research lobby began to move onto the offensive. Its members recognized that they would be able to win the parliamentary contest only if they could convince enough people that embryo research would generate major benefits of value to society at large.[26] They chose to place particular emphasis, as we have seen, on the prevention of disability, a topic which had been used with considerable success in the 1960s to promote the cause of abortion reform. But they had become aware that this topic had to be handled with great caution during the second half of the 1980s in order to ensure that fears about genetic engineering were not further exacerbated.

The pro-research lobby accomplished its task of collective persuasion by arguing that the scientists engaged in embryo research could greatly reduce the frequency of genetic disorders without developing techniques that involved the replacement or alteration of human genes. The crucial benefit to be derived from embryo research was identified as the capacity to enable couples who were likely to transmit genetic disability to choose to have a healthy IVF embryo implanted in the potential mother's womb.[27] This kind of procedure, it was stressed, did not change the embryo's genetic endowment and should be regarded, not as interference with the natural order, but merely as a way of improving the normal processes of embryonic wastage and natural selection.[28] Furthermore, it was argued, if embryo researchers were allowed to continue their work, they would actually make genetic engineering redundant. In the passage below, this point is emphasized by a leading embryologist who was also an active member of Progress.

Some people argue that any work of this kind is the thin end of the wedge, and will lead inevitably to the application of genetic engineering to humans. The reverse is true. At the moment, it is impossible to replace a defective gene with a normal one. Any attempt at such 'gene therapy' would introduce more genetic problems than it solved. One day it might become feasible. But it would still be pointless to attempt gene therapy if we have effective methods of preimplantation diagnosis. Every 'at risk' couple produces an abundance of unaffected sperm and eggs as well as affected ones. All that we need are ways to tell which is which.[29]

The idea of achieving genetic control by means of preimplantation diagnosis combined with selective screening of IVF embryos was rhetorically powerful because it seemed to offer the same therapeutic benefits as the more intrusive techniques of gene replacement, without transgressing the ultimate moral barrier to which all sides were committed. By the end of the sequence of debates, the majority of parliamentarians had accepted scientists' promises that these morally acceptable techniques would soon begin to generate major advances in the prevention of genetic disease. In some instances, the claims of the pro-research lobby became wildly exaggerated by lay enthusiasts who were inclined to credit embryo research and genetic screening with almost magical powers. Nonetheless, as we can see in the following passage, even the most ardent parliamentary advocates of embryo research were determined to make absolutely sure that these powers were not misused and that scientists would never be allowed to stray into forbidden areas:

Families carrying the gene of handicap may have a chance of healthy children as a result of research. How can we deny them that chance? Would it not be a good thing if the haemophilia gene was to vanish and if muscular dystrophy became a thing of the past? . . . I am not just speaking here of the most obvious diseases or the tragic diseases that have been described so graphically and in such moving terms tonight. I know that I speak for thousands of asthmatics when I say that if and when it is possible to avoid passing on our asthma to our children . . . we will give thanks to God and to those who carry out research which may some day make that possible . . . All research that leads to good ends could in the wrong hands be turned to evil . . . That is why I want to vote for strict controls and for the statutory licensing authority. That is why I regard this research as different. The law must be involved because the research is too important to be left to the doctors.[30]

The majority of parliamentarians finally decided to allow scientists to experiment on the so-called 'pre-embryo' and to develop techniques for selective implantation of healthy and defective embryos. But such research was seen as pressing very close to the limits of permissible conduct and, therefore, as requiring constant surveillance and regulation from outside. Thus parliamentarians insisted, without exception, that embryo research would have to be strictly controlled along the lines recommended by the Warnock Committee, in order to ensure that scientists would be unable to use relatively mature human embryos for experimental purposes or to interfere directly with the genetic structure of individual human organisms.

Those who spoke publicly on behalf of the scientific community had always maintained that there was no real danger of research on human embryos running out of control. However, the pro-research lobby had accepted, from the time of the debates over the Powell Bill, that there was no chance of obtaining parliamentary approval for such research without external regulation. As a result, those responsible for the organized campaign in support of embryo research had consistently supported the recommendations of the Warnock Report in favour of the creation of a statutory licensing authority. It had been made clear, therefore, well before the final parliamentary decision, that there was no disagreement between the scientific community and the lay supporters of embryo research about the need for legal and administrative mechanisms of control over the conduct of embryo research. In the words of Lord Jellicoe, head of the MRC, the scientists engaged in research involving human embryos would not merely comply with the Government's legislative proposals, but would actively welcome the introduction of a system of formal restraint and regulation which would bring to an end the current uncertainty:

I hope that the statutory licensing authority will be established in the near future. The regulatory regime proposed by the government would have – and I should like to say this very deliberately – the firm backing of my colleagues and myself in the Medical Research Council. As my noble and learned friend Lord Rawlinson observed in our debate over three years ago, this is too important a matter to be left to scientists. I agree. Funnily enough so do the scientists.[31]

The legislative proposal welcomed here by Lord Jellicoe was essentially that control over those morally sensitive aspects of embryo research identified in the Warnock Report and in subsequent parliamentary debate would be vested in an independent organization, with substantial lay membership, which would report to, and would ultimately be responsible to, Parliament. In the Government Bill, the necessary administrative apparatus was set up to license, monitor and regulate embryo research; the legitimate goals to be pursued by those active in embryo research were laid out; the nature of the biological material to be used was specified; various areas of potential experimentation were identified as illegal; and heavy penalties were introduced to encourage compliance with its requirements.[32] In confining embryo research in these ways, the Bill created a restricted social space in which legitimate scientific inquiry using human entities produced by means of IVF could be continued and, at the same time, contained. The dual purpose of the Bill was to make research possible in this morally difficult area, whilst ensuring that certain fundamental moral requirements, which were implicit in the details of the legislation, remained intact.

For most parliamentarians, the safe passage of the Government Bill meant that embryo research was finally under external control and that there was no need for further anxiety. But many of those who had participated in the long process of moral appraisal remained unconvinced and deeply disturbed about the future. For them, parliamentary approval of embryo research marked, not the resolution of a passing legislative difficulty, but an ominous shift in the balance of power between science and society which would have lasting repercussions in the years to come.

Those who say that this full-stop sized miniblob is not a human being must answer as to which part of the description it is to which they object – 'being' or 'human'. It is a being. Its nature and habits are known and we are talking about it. It is also alive and is made of human cells, not those of any other animal or plant. If it was not human you would not want it for research, and if it was not human no one would mind you having it for research . . . Licensing embryo research would be the beginning of a very slippery slope indeed. It is the threshold. After the first license to experiment on the undeniably human, the door is open.[33]

Many parliamentarians, particularly within the Conservative Party, still agreed with this speaker. These Members continued to insist that the use of human embryos was fundamentally immoral and that parliamentary approval of this form of immoral conduct would slowly but surely change the processes through which scientists gained access to, and use of, human organisms. In the long term, they argued, this would corrupt and degrade our basic beliefs about what it is to be human. However, by the end of the sequence of debates, this negative assessment of embryo research had ceased to be dominant. The pro-research lobby had succeeded in persuading the majority of parliamentarians to adopt a much more optimistic vision of a compliant community of licensed investigators delivering massive therapeutic benefit in a manner that furthered society's humane objectives whilst preserving its fundamental morality. This representation of embryo research, guaranteed by the authority of the scientific establishment, appealed directly to that subtle combination of progressive and conservative ideals that defines the middle ground of British politics. The pro-research lobby succeeded because the majority both of Labour progressives and of Conservative moderates were unable to resist a programme of controlled scientific development which, so they believed, had been shown to offer substantial social progress without requiring any significant alteration to social values or to essential social relationships.

5

Embryos in the news

During the passage of the Human Fertilization and Embryology Bill, the media of mass communication relayed the various views expressed in Parliament to the public at large and commented on the issues involved. Because opinion remained deeply divided among the wider population, and because the outcome of the parliamentary process seemed uncertain to the very end, embryo research continued to be newsworthy until the final vote had been taken. Those for, as well as those against, embryo research attempted to use the media to influence public opinion and, thereby, to incline wavering MPs in their favour.

Both sides had previously commissioned surveys of public opinion and had used the results to strengthen their recommendations that embryo research should, or should not, be allowed to continue. But as the debate entered its last phase, the opponents of embryo research appeared to be losing the battle of the polls. This point was emphasized in Parliament by the advocates of such research.[1] Some of those arguing for the prohibition of embryo research still insisted that the public was on their side. However, in order to make this assertion at all convincing, they had to try to show that the pollsters' measurements of opinion were inaccurate. Other opponents of embryo research accepted that there had been a swing in public opinion, but alleged that this was due to the fact that many ordinary people had been misled by the pro-research lobby's public relations campaign and by the biased treatment of the topic in the media: 'Those of us who have tried to follow the topic closely as it has developed over the winter since it was debated in [the Lords] were struck by the deluge of one-sided publicity, not only this weekend in quality newspapers or on behalf of one programme in one hospital . . . '[2]

This assessment of media coverage of embryo research during the final stage of parliamentary debate is supported by the evidence. In the press, for example, presentations in favour of embryo research outnumbered those opposed to such research by a ratio of five to two.[3] This pronounced imbalance frustrated the critics of embryo research and led to the accusation of media bias. From their perspective, of course, any firm endorsement of embryo research necessarily involved some kind of misrepresentation. Thus, the widespread and enthusiastic advocacy on behalf of embryo research to be found in the media during the final phase of debate was seen by them as a clear indication that the media were not dealing impartially with this issue, but were being improperly manipulated to serve the interests of their opponents. On the other hand, from the point of view of those active in the pro-research lobby, their domination of the media was a just reward for their sustained efforts as well as a necessary part of their strategy for gaining parliamentary approval for controlled research on human embryos.

The image of embryo research in the press

The essence of the case for embryo research presented in the newspapers is evident in the headlines used to attract potential readers:

> **A vote to diminish suffering** *Guardian*
> **I cried when I saved mother from another doomed baby** *Today*
> **When science stops pain** *Evening Standard*
> **Wife who found joy backs embryo research** *Daily Mail*
> **In step with the quick march of science** *Sunday Times*
> **A ray of hope for millions** *The Independent*

As these headlines suggest, discussions of embryo research in the press repeatedly described how research of this kind would lead to more control over pain, further relief from suffering, more frequent personal fulfilment and, hence, to greater joy and happiness. The primary message in these newspaper presentations was that the use of science-based techniques offered hope to many unfortunate women of a better reproductive future. This message of hope was regularly conveyed and reinforced by means of highly personal narratives.[4] In these narratives, dramatic improvements in women's experience of childbirth were linked to the new technology of reproduction which was, in turn, linked to prior research. Thus the 'joy' of an infertile wife who became pregnant through IVF or the 'ecstasy' of a woman implanted with a healthy, instead of a 'doomed', embryo were used to display to the public the hope inherent in embryo research and to encourage parliamentary support for the continuation of such research. The *Daily Mail*, for example, in an article offering 'hope for thousands', concluded:

'If Parliament votes next week to ban further embryo research, other women who are carriers of genetic diseases may not have the chance of having a healthy baby granted to these mothers.'[5]

Articles that were organized around the joy experienced by specific women focused on the benefits produced by medical techniques that already existed, such as IVF or preimplantation diagnosis. These stories were used, however, to make the point that new techniques would be developed, and that further benefits would soon follow, if embryo research was allowed to continue. This line of argument was explored more fully in articles in which the merits of embryo research were considered in more general terms. These discussions frequently went far beyond the present achievements of science, as authors presented strong claims about the long-term consequences of research on human embryos. In these texts, the future accomplishments of embryo research become strangely tangible. It is as if, even though the researchers have yet to carry out the necessary experiments, the eventual findings of scientific research are already known and its benefits are waiting to be voted into existence.

This style of argumentation can be seen in the following passages which have been taken from newspaper items published on the day of the final debate in the House of Commons:

Tonight MPs face a decision which could change the personal and family lives of millions of people. A vote to ban embryo research would mean anxiety and heartbreak for families which are carriers of genetic conditions . . . It would mean less hope of having a much-wanted child for couples experiencing the frustrations of infertility . . . Much benefit can accrue from research . . . One in seven of all couples experience difficulty in having children. If they are to be helped to the maximum of medical ability, such research must continue . . . In the near future . . . screening techniques will identify genetic defects irrespective of sex, and enable families to avoid transmitting disability if they so desire. With such enormous hope on the horizon, how on earth can Parliament seriously consider banning such research, and taking away from people a choice of avoiding disability?   *The Independent*[6]

Today there can be no doubt about the enormous happiness brought by *in vitro* fertilization to thousands of infertile couples . . . There is no way to all this happiness without research on embryos . . . Research on the human embryo is essential if we are to improve the treatment of infertility; to find out why some embryos grow disastrously and simply degenerate; to find out why some embryos never implant into their mothers. It will tell us why embryo cells and cancer cells have so much in common and how those abnormal genes which can lead to such terrible handicaps start on their destructive path . . . For the sake of thousands of unborn children, I implore our MPs to take the right decision today and to support embryo research.

Daily Mail[7]

These texts move beyond particular narratives and individual examples of the benefits of research to bring out its broader significance. The reader is assured that the technical advances and the enormous happiness already achieved can be taken as guarantees of further scientific achievements, and hence of much more happiness, yet to come. Scientific research is treated as an area of human conduct where one can speak with confidence of what the future has in store. In such articles we are told, not only what science will accomplish, but also what the social consequences will be. For example, the item from *The Independent* informs us that the development of genetic screening techniques will enable families to avoid transmitting disability if they so desire. The power of these texts derives from the implicit assumption that their authors can foresee the medical and social future by reference to the future shape of science.

Embryo research is justified in articles of this kind by means of an evocation of a better future which will be experienced, not just by a few fortunate individuals, but by anyone who wishes to take advantage of the new reproductive technologies. In the world constructed in these texts, relief from suffering and an increase in joy and happiness follow unproblematically from the advance of scientific knowledge. There is no mention in these presentations of the massive changes in clinical practice or the great expansion in artificially assisted pregnancy that would be required in order to make screening techniques available to all families at risk of genetic disability. Similarly, no consideration is given to the possibility that people's definitions of 'genetic risk' might alter in response to the new technology, thereby greatly enlarging popular demand for genetic screening. In other words, these representations seek to justify the continuation of embryo research by projecting its presumed results into a radically simplified future in which each scientific achievement leads directly, without encountering any significant obstacles, to a substantial increase in social benefit.

Scientific research, of course, is frequently justified by reference to the social benefits it is likely to generate.[8] In this respect, the case presented for embryo research in the press was not unusual. It was simply one more example of a new area of scientific endeavour being depicted in terms of a public rhetoric expressing the confident expectation of a better future through the application of science. However, the advocacy in favour of embryo research during the final stages of the parliamentary debate seems to have been an extreme instance of this kind of rhetoric in the sense that so little attention was given by its supporters in the press either to scientific or to practical uncertainties.

One reason for this lack of moderation in the campaign on behalf of embryo research was that those involved were, at least at the outset, fighting for survival against a well-organized and long-established opposition.[9] The arguments they presented on behalf of embryo research, in Parliament and in the press, were designed to redress this political and ideological imbalance. In these circumstances, it was natural for the pro-research lobby to avoid making any admissions of weakness which might be exploited by their opponents. The central aim of the pro-research campaign was to defeat these opponents by placing unswerving emphasis on the use of scientific research to engender various kinds of therapeutic advance.[10] In short, the presentation of the case for embryo research in the press and elsewhere during the final phase of debate was oversimplified and one-sided at least partly because it was a reaction against the organized attack upon embryo research with which the public debate had begun.[11]

Mothers, babies and embryo research

The fundamental benefit cited to justify embryo research and the techniques of assisted reproduction was, of course, that they would help women to have babies. In this respect, the successes of the new reproductive technologies have been considerable. Nevertheless, it is acknowledged that the failure rate, for example, of IVF, remains disturbingly high.[12] As a result, most women who use the science-based techniques of assisted reproduction do not give birth. Thus it is possible to tell stories of failure and disappointment about assisted reproduction as well as stories of fulfilment and success.[13] During the period under study, however, the press concentrated narrowly on happily married women who had been made pregnant or who had already given birth with the help of the new technologies. The much greater number of women for whom the technology had failed, and for whom there may have been more suffering than joy, were almost completely ignored. If such women had been given greater prominence, they would have tended to undermine the standardized progressive story-line, in both its personal and its more general forms. Consequently, although ordinary women were present and textually active in many newspaper presentations, their contributions were carefully selected and controlled in accordance with the guiding image of a beneficent convergence between science, technology and conventional motherhood.

This image is evident in the way in which women were visually outnumbered in the newspapers by their offspring. During the final phase of debate, there were more than twice as many photographs of children and babies as there were photographs of women.[14] This visual imbalance reflected women's relationship to children in these texts. For women were present only as potential or actual bearers of children. The ultimate concern of those stories in which women appeared was not women as such, but the babies that they might be able to produce. For instance, just before the final Commons debate, the *Daily Mirror* published a seven-page feature in praise of embryo research, IVF and other techniques of assisted reproduction. It was entitled **BABY SPECIAL**.[15] Whereas the case against embryo research emphasized the harm it did to minute, invisible 'unborn children', the case for such research focused on the production of real, full-scale, visible children. By the time of the final parliamentary debates, unborn children had been displaced from the media by a throng of happy, smiling babies.

The *Mirror's* **BABY SPECIAL** was largely composed of pictures of such babies accompanied by their stories. These stories employed a simple structure built around the assisted production of a 'baby without blemish'. This structure has three basic elements. The first is a married woman who has been unable to bear a (healthy) child, but who is now pregnant or has recently given birth to a (healthy) child as a result of IVF or some similar technique. This component is used to create a contrast between the mother's (and/or other women's) previous experience of distress, frustration or anguish, and her present state of unqualified joy. Finally the arrival, or the expected arrival, of the baby and the happiness that follows are attributed to the use of science-based technology.

This structure is exemplified in the two following cases taken from the **BABY SPECIAL**.

Suzanne Buckley was just 16 when gynaecologists told her bluntly she would never have a child. They were wrong. Today, at 29, the once heartbroken teenager is the doting mum of an eight-month-old son. But she knows it could never have happened but for the skill of doctors and the generosity of an unknown woman who donated a perfect egg. Suzanne suffers from Turner's Syndrome. Her ovaries have not formed properly . . . 'I eventually got a place at King's College and was put on hormone treatment' . . . The first implant failed – but the second was a success. 'When I was told I cried and cried. It was the happiest moment of my life.'

Even now, two years later, test-tube mum Katy Shaw can hardly express her joy at the moment she learned she was pregnant. 'You can't really explain how good you feel', she says, 'because those are the words you dreamed about hearing for so long. For Chris and me it seemed like a miracle' . . . Teacher Katy, 34, and husband, Chris, paid [for treatment] at King's College Hospital, London, in their bid for a baby of their own. After five years and seven attempts their efforts were rewarded. Katy fell pregnant. And today she is the proud and happy mother of . . . 20-month-old twin boys . . . 'I have what doctors call "unexplained infertility" and I'm told its quite common,' Katy says . . . 'That is why research must continue.'

The contrast between joy and suffering around which such texts are organized requires the arrival of a baby. Furthermore, it is necessary for the baby to be free from major defects; as in the case of Suzanne Buckley, the egg must be presumed to be 'perfect'. If this were not so, the mother's joy might be tempered by further suffering and the meaning of her experience would become equivocal. Thus, the woman's contribution to this kind of story is entirely derivative. She can be given textual space only insofar as she longs for a baby, has suffered on the baby's behalf and has eventually, with the scientists' help, succeeded in bearing a baby. The recent or imminent arrival of a baby without blemish is essential because this is a story of hope. The baby symbolizes hope for a better future through the power of science. Without the baby, there is no hope and no story. Without the baby, there is no role for the woman to perform.

This narrative structure, which was widely used in the pro-research press campaign, was constructed by means of a simple formula designed in accordance with the requirements of the rhetoric of hope. This does not mean that the stories told in this way were false or that they were consciously manipulative. There can be no doubt that contributors to the media drew upon semantic contrasts and narrative components that were used by many childless women and by other participants in assisted reproduction.[16] In this sense, the media accounts were true to their sources. Nevertheless, alternative story-lines and rhetorical vocabularies were available and could have been used more frequently by the press to provide a richer and more varied appraisal of these new developments in biomedical science.

Let us consider an example. One of the handful of critical articles to appear during the final stage of debate focused on a technique known as GIFT (gamete intra-fallopian transfer).[17] This technique was described in the article as having the advantage of being cheaper than IVF and, therefore, as being likely to become more widely used, but also as having the disadvantage of increasing the incidence of multiple births. In order to illustrate the kind of problems that could occur with this technique, the story of a particular 'infertile woman' was told. In this story, the standard contrast between present joy and past suffering was dramatically overturned. The woman's dream of having a healthy baby was seen to have been transformed into a nightmare as the GIFT technique made her pregnant with quadruplets. As a result of her multiple pregnancy, the woman gave birth prematurely. The consequence was that two of her babies died quickly and the other two remained seriously ill and confined to hospital.

This story, like the standard pro-research narrative, dealt with the personal consequences of assisted reproduction. But it was constructed around a cruel reversal of the customary story-line and moved away from the simplistic rhetoric of hope towards a more complex assessment of embryo research and its associated techniques. The story of this mother and of her gravely impaired babies tells of an alternative future where the new technologies may produce harm as well as good, where the cost of medical techniques can be as important as their clinical reliability and where the practical consequences for NHS neonatal units may be devastating.[18]

It was, then, possible to tell quite a different kind of story which drew attention to the occurrence of technological failure and extreme personal distress, and to the difficulties arising from the introduction of modern techniques of assisted reproduction into the medical bureaucracy. It would also have been possible to write about the experiences of women who had not produced babies. In the months following the birth of Louise Brown in 1978, the *Daily Mirror* had published several articles telling the stories of women for whom IVF had failed and commenting critically on the activities of Edwards and Steptoe.[19] But, as the parliamentary debate drew to a close, the *Mirror*, like most other newspapers, chose to celebrate the achievements of assisted reproduction and to ignore what could have been seen as its failures.

In view of the low take-home-baby rate of the techniques of assisted reproduction, stories of failure and disappointment would have been more representative of women's actual experiences than the standard success story that pervaded the media. Even if we were to imagine a future in which implantation of embryos by means of IVF and related techniques had become as efficient as the natural processes of reproduction in human populations, there would still be two failures for every successful pregnancy.[20] In other words, not only is it the case that the great majority of artificially assisted women do not give birth, but it seems likely that this may always be so. Thus, although the 'arrival of the baby without blemish' is one relevant narrative structure for embryo research and its technologies, there is another, perhaps even more appropriate, story-line which might might be called 'the disappointed woman'. Such a story-line could have been used in the newspapers to argue that this whole approach to the reduction of childlessness was fundamentally defective and that scientific research should be primarily concerned with identifying, and eliminating, the *causes* of infertility and thereby bringing relief to a much larger proportion of infertile women.[21] However, the narrative of 'the disappointed woman' was never used in the press during the period under study, even though this narrative had been employed earlier to express doubts about the test-tube baby project and even though there must have been women able to tell this story in every infertility clinic.[22]

These observations should not be taken to imply that women who have failed to benefit from their use of the techniques of assisted reproduction would necessarily condemn embryo research. There is evidence to show that many women in this situation continue to support research and its associated technologies.[23] Nevertheless, their personal stories would inevitably have been very different from the customary tale of the arrival of the 'baby without blemish' and would have required a more complex appraisal of the benefits and disadvantages of embryo research. Their absence from the media was a significant omission which worked to the short-term advantage of the pro-research campaign by promoting a simplistic, yet powerful, image of the natural beneficence of science.

Narrative control in the media

Although the narrative of 'the disappointed woman' was never used by the press during the final period of parliamentary debate, there was opposition to embryo research which emphasized the negative consequences of the pursuit of scientific knowledge in this area. Contributions of this kind in the newspapers were similar in content to many of the formal speeches against embryo research in Parliament. In these critical articles, scientists' motives and use of technical language were questioned; attention was drawn to scientists' supposed unwillingness to respect the sanctity of life; accusations were made that the benefits of research were being grossly exaggerated in the course of a crude public relations campaign; and prophetic warnings were delivered about the approach of an age of scientific barbarism. The following passage provides one illustration of this 'rhetoric of fear' in operation in the press:

HIDEOUS STRENGTH
It was an evil day for our country and the world when MPs voted to allow experiments on the human embryo 'under strict conditions', as the saying is. But nobody should be surprised at this triumph of 'the spirit of scientific inquiry'. It is the dominant spirit of our age; its power over the public mind and the minds of MPs is overwhelming. For weeks now, in preparation for the Parliamentary debate, the campaign for 'embryo research' has been rumbling away in the 'media' . . . The argument which seeks to shame us all into compliance with the enormities of embryo research, to abandon all previous taboos, all previous ideas of what is right and wrong, lawful and unlawful, and even all human common sense, runs like this: that such experiments will eventually relieve certain kinds of human suffering. There are many people who sincerely believe this. But there seems to be no evidence, even in strictly scientific terms, that they are right. What scientists are really after is absolute freedom for experimental science as an end in itself, on the principle that because a thing is scientifically possible it must be done, and no law or custom must ever prevent it. This principle has already brought terrible, previously unheard of evils into the world. Today it seems irresistible. But all is not lost. For all the overweening arrogance of our perverted science . . . it cannot last for ever.

Daily Telegraph[24]

In the parliamentary context this powerful condemnation, rejecting the basic claims advanced on behalf of embryo research and warning of its fearful consequences, would have been one among many similar statements. In the newspapers of the period, it is almost unique.[25] Furthermore, not only did opposition to embryo research occupy little space in the newspapers, it also relied entirely on the kind of generalized invective employed in the passage quoted above. Unlike the rhetoric of hope, which was repeatedly embodied in numerous variations on the 'baby without blemish' story, the counter-rhetoric of fear remained curiously removed from accounts of ordinary people's experience. As a result, criticisms of embryo research in the press lacked the personal dimension that supplemented, and provided support for, the strong claims made concerning the future benefits of such research. The attainment of this monopoly over the kind of emotive personal story on which the popular press depends was a major tactical victory for the pro-research lobby.

One reason for the virtual absence of opposition narratives from the press was that the media obtained most of their stories about assisted reproduction and embryo research from the major infertility clinics in London. These clinics furnished a regular series of heartwarming human-interest stories ideally suited to the pro-research rhetoric of medical advance and personal fulfilment through science-based technology. Because most stories originated in this way, scientists were almost always central figures in the personal narratives about assisted reproduction that appeared in the newspapers. In many instances, the public presentation of these success stories was clearly initiated by the scientists involved. Furthermore, it is clear that certain major stories – for example, those dealing with screening for inherited diseases by means of sexual selection – were released to the press in a calculated fashion at critical points in the parliamentary process. It seems reasonable, therefore, to infer that the imbalance between pro-research and anti-research narratives in the media was largely a consequence of scientists' presence as gatekeepers and their ability to regulate the flow of material, to a considerable degree, in accordance with their own interests and their own definition of the situation.

In practice, a very small group of prominent scientists acted as intermediaries between the public at large and those people who had experienced the science-based technologies of assisted reproduction. These scientists made available to the public, via the media of mass communication, a sequence of women through whom the value of embryo research was revealed. By means of the stories told about these women, science was shown to contribute in a direct, personal fashion to family life, both now and in a better world to come.

Joyful Debbie Edwards yesterday cradled the hopes of thousands of couples in her arms. Her new-born twins, Natalie and Danielle, are the world's first babies to have their sex determined in a test tube. The breakthrough, pioneered by Professor Robert Winston at the Hammersmith Hospital in London, is the first step in a revolutionary treatment which doctors hope will eventually wipe out all hereditary diseases . . . Mr Edwards, 35, who was with his wife throughout the birth, said: 'To us, it doesn't matter that they're a world first. They are the perfect family we have been waiting for.'   *Daily Mail*[26]

Many of the stories appearing in the newspapers centred around the activities of Professor Winston. This was partly because Winston was the head of a major infertility centre and partly because he was also the most publicly visible member of Progress. During this period, Winston acted as the main representative of the embryo research community. As a result, like his patients, his personal life was examined in some detail. He was shown to be, not only a dedicated scientist, but also a loving husband and father whose overriding aim was to help others to enjoy the kind of domestic bliss that characterized his own family relationships.

It is 8am when the first of dozens of phone calls disturbs Professor Winston's breakfast at his north London home . . . Through his pioneering work at the Infertility Unit of Hammersmith Hospital, Professor Winston has brought happiness to countless thousands . . . He has brought to the embryo debate the gritty determination that is the hallmark of all aspects of his life. The pond and waterfall in a corner of the garden were dug by him, his proud wife Lira reveals. 'Has he told you all the things he's good at? He built the rabbit-run and he's brilliant at icing birthday cakes,' she says. Winston himself is characteristically modest . . . He adores his children but feels guilty about neglecting them through pressure of work . . . They, together with the thousands of parents to whom he has given new hope, need no persuading that here is a great man.   *Today*[27]

Both sides in the embryo debate were able to engage effectively in generalized dispute about the rights and wrongs of embryo research and its consequences for the family. But, among the contestants over the future of embryo research, scientists alone succeeded in being depicted in the media, through the figure of Professor Winston, both as embodying the ideal of proper family life and as enabling people who had previously been excluded from normal domesticity to create happy families of their own.

The power of the pro-research campaign

We cannot observe directly the success of the pro-research campaign in influencing public opinion.[28] Nevertheless, it is possible to obtain some indication of its persuasive power by comparing two editorials published in the *Evening Standard*. The first of these appeared on 9 February 1990, shortly after the final debate about embryo research in the Lords. In this instance, the editorial voice spoke unreservedly against the continuation of research. In characteristic anti-research fashion, scientists' morality was questioned, their misuse of language was denounced and reference to the Nazi scientist Dr Josef Mengele was used to convey the depths of their depravity.

THE SANCTITY OF HUMAN LIFE

Conceptus. Pre-embryo. Primitive streak. Fetus. These are some of the Newspeak words which are used nowadays to describe a child in the earliest stages of his or her development . . . There is only one minor distinction between the life of a human being who has been born and the life of a recently-conceived child in the womb or the test-tube: the former is visibly human and the latter, though no less human, is invisible. This distinction is one of appearances only. It is the sole basis for regarding Dr Mengele, whose obsessive desire to extend the frontiers of medical knowledge led him to repudiate the humanity of the victims whom he slaughtered, as more obviously culpable than the medical experimenter of today, whose desire to discover ways of preventing genetic disease is honourable but whose failure to respect the humanity of the little ones upon whom they wish to experiment is, to say the least, regrettable. 'Medical ethics' is now a contradiction in terms . . . Every human being, however small, is entitled to his or her chance of life and nobody, however actually honourable his motives or potentially useful his researches, should be allowed to tamper with that precious life.   *Evening Standard*[29]

In the quotation below, taken from an editorial published five weeks later, a significant evaluative change has occurred. In this second editorial, the medical benefits of embryo research as well as its basic legitimacy have come to be clearly, although somewhat grudgingly, admitted. Condemnation has given way to acceptance and the expression of hope for a better future. Of particular significance is the fact that this moral reappraisal has been directly linked to the stories of three women who had been implanted with genetically screened embryos in Professor Winston's clinic.

WHEN SCIENCE STOPS PAIN

Embryo research is tinkering with the sanctity of human life and strict laws will always be required to prevent the perversion of advanced techniques. But today there is news of medical advances in this field which represent the other, more acceptable side of the coin. Doctors can now identify the sex of test-tube babies before they are implanted in the womb of the mother-to-be. This is important because it allows parents-to-be whose family histories reveal disorders among boys to implant only girls. Three women who took part in the Hammersmith Hospital experiment are now carrying healthy, female babies. Professor Winston estimates that his team may be able to treat in a year as many as 100 women who have grounds for anxiety about the sex of the child they are carrying . . . Arguments about science's potential for evil cannot be used to stifle research, or to uninvent techniques for which there is a   demand. The research of Professor Winston and his team has brought hope to people who face the dilemma of wanting a child but knowing there is a 50-50 chance that it will be born severely disabled. In the past such people had two choices: they could decide against having children or they could take a chance that they would not be damaged. Now we rejoice that science has provided a better one.   *Evening Standard*[30]

This editorial reassessment seems to be a direct response to the story of the three pregnant women that was announced by Winston to the press just five days before the final Commons vote. It is a clear example of how the release of material of this kind was carefully regulated. In addition, it shows how powerful such stories were, not only in furnishing resources for the case in favour of embryo research, but also in weakening the arguments against. The essential case for research was physically embodied in the smiling, happily pregnant women who appeared that day, chastely embraced by Winston, on the front pages of the popular daily papers. These joyful women were symbols of the countless happy families to come. Against this optimistic celebration of science and the family, the opponents of embryo research had little to offer apart from what had come to appear as rather hysterical warnings about unspecified horrors waiting further down the slippery slope. The marked editorial shift contained in the quotations above is an illustration of the way in which the opposition case more or less disappeared from the media under the pressure of the narrative material strategically released by members of the pro-research lobby. This success in the media may well have had a major impact on public opinion concerning embryo research and assisted reproduction; and thereby on the actions of the decision-makers in Parliament.

We have seen in this chapter that the parliamentary accusation of 'media bias' in relation to embryo research was justified in the sense that, by the final phase of debate, the case in favour of research on human embryos did dominate the media. This accusation was an understandable response to the oversimplified, idealized rhetoric employed on behalf of embryo research; and to the fact that this rhetoric was remarkably effective. The charge of bias, however, must have appeared disingenuous to the supporters of embryo research. For the shape of their own campaign had been formed in direct reaction to the heated denunciations of embryo research with which the debate had started. The extreme, unqualified affirmation of the benefits of embryo research by its advocates was but a mirror image of the total condemnation that the Warnock Committee's cautious endorsement of research on human embryos had elicited from so many parliamentarians and members of the wider public.

The supporters of embryo research won the public debate, as well as the debate in Parliament, because they managed eventually to create a simple, yet powerful, pro-research rhetoric which combined the authority of science with moving personal testimony; because they exerted a pronounced influence upon the flow of commentary and narrative material in the media during the final, decisive phase of debate; because they succeeded in gaining widespread publicity for a series of convincing examples of the benefits of embryo research; and because they were able to link their case directly to conventional family values.

6

Women and men

Shortly after the vote in the Upper House in February 1990 in favour of embryo research, a female contributor to the *Sunday Correspondent* pointed out that the fate of embryo research would finally be decided in the House of Commons by 607 men and 42 women. The author complained that it was inappropriate and unjust that a legislative decision that would have such a significant impact on women's experiences of childbirth should be taken mainly by men.[1] A similar concern over the parliamentary dominance of men was present among women in Parliament. Several female Labour MPs had protested, during the opening phase of debate, that the central issues were being defined largely by men and that women's opinions were being ignored. These speakers maintained that women's view of human reproduction and of embryo research tended to differ from that of men; and that women's intimate and continual involvement in the reproductive process would enable them, if they were given the opportunity, to make a particularly significant contribution to parliamentary discussion of these matters. In passages such as those quoted below, taken from the Commons debate in February 1985, female speakers expressed their frustration at women's limited representation in Parliament and at what they depicted as the failure of the male majority to appreciate the potential value of women's distinctive testimony:

In some sense [the opening speaker] has put his finger on the essence of the debate in assuming that it concerns the dignity of man. However, it also concerns the dignity of women, and that should not be forgotten. I am not being frivolous. At the beginning of the debate, Mr Speaker announced that more than 40 hon. Gentlemen wished to speak, and in so doing ignored the fact that there were several women in the House who also wanted to contribute to the debate.[2]

I wish to amplify the point made [above] by my hon. Friend Ms Richardson. Women understand these matters in a way that men do not, because they deal with them in their daily life. They menstruate, conceive or do not conceive, worry about whether they will have children . . . and so on. Women are more familiar with the subject, whereas men set it up as a set of moral principles and logical constructs. Women know that thousands of conceptuses are wasted by nature . . . Nature has organized fertility wastefully.   Conceptuses are destroyed month by month, through miscarriages, the use of the coil and for all sorts of reasons. Men must face that.[3]

The claims made in statements such as these were not disinterested. They were intended to give special weight to the views of those women who spoke in favour of embryo research. At the same time, however, they raise a number of interesting questions about the possible significance of gender in the parliamentary process whereby embryo research came to be officially ratified. Four such questions will be explored in this chapter. Firstly, to what extent was women's involvement in reproduction taken to be relevant to the topic of embryo research? Secondly, how far did women's contributions to parliamentary debate on this topic differ from those of men? Thirdly, how far did women and men differ in their support for embryo research? Finally, what rhetorical use was made of the notion that women have a special understanding of the moral issues arising in relation to embryo research?[4]

These questions will be addressed by means of close examination of the final phase of parliamentary debate. Detailed comparisons will be made between the contributions of male and female speakers in the eight-hour session in the House of Lords in December 1989 with which discussion of the Government Bill began; and in the seven-hour session in the House of Commons in April 1990 that gave final parliamentary approval to research on human IVF embryos.[5] Although the decision-making procedure was dominated by men, a number of women did speak in these debates. In the Lords, there were thirty-eight men and eleven women; in the Commons, there were seven women and twenty-four men.[6] Because most speakers and the great majority of the audience were male, let us begin by considering what men had to say.

A discourse of the embryo

The final debate in the House of Commons was opened by the Secretary of State for Health. The Secretary of State began by identifying the central issue of the debate as 'whether or not to allow the kind of research being done now on human embryos to continue'.[7] He then undertook a review of the arguments proposed for and against research by various interested parties. In clarifying the case in favour of research, he spoke as follows:

I think that the researchers all say that it would be irresponsible for doctors to replace in the womb fertilized human eggs that had been subjected to novel procedures or tests, for these might themselves lead to abnormality. They say that to use the mother as part of the research, and then to put in an embryo which has been subjected to research and might have been made abnormal by research, would be unacceptable.[8]

In this passage, the Secretary of State acknowledged that women are regularly involved in embryo research. He seems to have taken it for granted that 'mothers' are 'used' as part of that research. Given that the Secretary of State's task was to establish the frame of reference for the debate, it might have been reasonable to expect that the experimental use of women would have been taken up as a major theme by subsequent contributors.

In fact, women's involvement in embryo research and in its associated technologies received very little attention, particularly from men, in either House. This can be shown by considering how frequently references were made in the two debates to 'women' or to 'mothers', and how these references were distributed. In the debate in the Lords in December 1989, only ten of the thirty-eight male speakers referred explicitly to women. In contrast, ten of the eleven female speakers did so. In the Commons, only eight out of twenty-four men explicitly mentioned women; whereas six out of the seven women did so. In short, the great majority of male contributors expressed their views on embryo research and the technologies of assisted reproduction, during these crucial debates, without direct reference to women's participation in the research or to the consequences for women of the new technologies.

Embryo research is not concerned exclusively with laboratory embryos. Its biological focus is the relationship between fertilized human eggs and the female bodies without which embryos are unable to develop. Most embryo research is closely linked to the design of techniques to assist women in the process of reproduction. In 1989, forty-one of the fifty-three licensed projects in Britain 'were devoted to discovering why IVF often fails and to improve the treatment of infertility'.[9] Work on the improvement of reproductive techniques necessarily depends on the sustained involvement of women.[10] In the parliamentary appraisal of embryo research, however, male speakers were much more concerned about human embryos than about women.

This concentration on the human embryo was established in the opening speeches by the Government representatives in both major debates under detailed consideration here. In the Commons, as we have seen, the issue presented for debate by the Secretary of State was not whether women should continue to be used for experimental purposes, but only whether embryos should continue to be used in this way. A similar definition of the main question to be resolved was furnished in the Lords. Indeed, in the Lord Chancellor's opening speech, which was repeatedly praised by subsequent speakers for its even-handedness, there were no explicit references at all to women; at least, to women as social actors. There was one brief mention of a 'woman's uterus'.[11] But the reference here was more to embryos than to women. For the point being made was that the human embryo has no prospect of becoming a person unless it implants in a uterus. The Lord Chancellor was concerned in this part of his speech, not with women as persons, but only with women as sites for the maturation of human embryos. In both opening speeches, therefore, women featured only insofar as they had some bearing on the physiology of human reproduction.

These two speeches, both by men, set the tone for the majority of male contributors. The passages below, the first from the Lords and the second from the Commons, illustrate how men were inclined to follow the example of the Government speakers in concentrating on the moral implications of the embryo's involvement in research:

The only issue I wish to deal with today is whether under supervision of the statutory licensing authority we should permit or prohibit research on the pre-embryo during the 14 days from fertilization.[12]

In spite of the apparent technical complexity of the matter, the fundamental issue is clear-cut and straightforward. I am glad that . . . the Secretary of State for Health highlighted that primary consideration. The simple issue is at what point in the interaction between the ovum and the sperm human life begins. Once human life has begun . . . can any form of experimentation on the material substance of that human life at any stage be either ethical or acceptable if it is not intended for the well-being, good and survival of that form of human life, however embryonic and elemental it may be?[13]

In the concise phrase of another male speaker: 'The subject of our debate is the embryonic human.'[14] The dominance of this view meant that the potential issue of women's involvement in research and assisted reproduction receded into the background as speaker after speaker based his appraisal of embryo research on his assessment of the humanity and proper treatment of the isolated early embryo. Acknowledgement of women's role in embryo research and in the new technologies could be said to be implicit in men's talk about IVF, embryo transfer, egg donation, and so on. But women's involvement was taken by most men to be unproblematic. The great majority of men seem to have assumed, as did the initial Government speakers, that the treatment of women, unlike the treatment of embryos, was in no need of careful, public scrutiny.

There remains, however, a substantial minority of men, one in three in the Commons and one in four in the Lords, who did make explicit reference to women in their formal speeches. The average number of explicit references to women by these men in the Commons was three. In the Lords, it was lower still. Thus, the issue of women's participation in research and assisted reproduction remained a subsidiary theme even among the members of this minority. Those men who mentioned women explicitly in the course of speeches in favour of embryo research consistently represented such research and its technologies as working to women's advantage. In so doing, they focused on the production of healthy babies and happy families. There are no examples of male supporters of embryo research drawing attention, in the two major debates under consideration here, to women's role as experimental subjects or exploring the possibility that the technology of assisted reproduction might have negative consequences for women.[15] Issues of this kind were raised only by the opponents of embryo research.

I am making a serious charge, and I would like to hear someone responsible in Government address the matter. I am advised that the use of such [fertility] drugs can cause serious problems for women. It is no more than treating women, as well as the human embryos used in research, as guinea pigs.[16]

IVF is inefficient, time-consuming and dangerous for women. It can lead to cysts, coagulation, strokes, heart problems, ovarian cancer and many other problems. Babies born from IVF have three times the rate of low birth weight, five times the spina bifida rate and four times the perinatal death rate.[17]

Such speakers, although they normally mentioned the disadvantages for babies or embryos as well as for women, appear in occasional passages of this kind to have been identifying women as independent agents with rights which need to be considered seriously alongside those of the embryo. However, the question of the potentially dangerous consequences arising for women from their involvement in research and in the new reproductive technologies was not taken up by other contributors. One reason for this may have been that, despite these brief references to women's problems, the main focus of opposition to embryo research was its threat to the rights of the embryo. Mention of women's difficulties was no more than a minor tactic within a broad strategy designed to safeguard the embryo by discrediting embryo research in every possible way. As a result, it tended to occur in passing as one of a list of accusations levelled at embryo research, after which speakers returned quickly to their main theme.

Because women's interests were not central to their case, male opponents of research sometimes seemed a little erratic in their treatment of this topic.

For example, Alan Amos, the speaker in the last quotation, emphasized there that IVF was dangerous for women. Elsewhere in his speech, however, he said: 'I am not and have never been against IVF, but I oppose the deliberate artificial creation of human life simply to destroy it.'[18] It seems to be implied here that the dangers for women of IVF were not, after all, terribly important. The critical issue for this man, as for most male critics of embryo research, was not the effects of IVF on women, but the emergence of a form of intervention in the process of reproduction that seemed to them to put in jeopardy the embryo's right to life. In his concluding words, Amos made this absolutely clear:

To allow human embryo research is to infringe the moral rule that we should not use others for our own needs. What use is the Hippocratic oath, the Helsinki declaration or any other definition of moral values, if the people whom we trust – doctors, scientists and politicians – constantly and persistently abuse their special positions and live the lie that the unborn child is not alive and is not human?[19]

These remarks bring us back to those rights and needs of the embryo that provided the essential point of reference for the majority of men's contributions to parliamentary debate on this topic. Whether they were Labour or Conservative, whether they spoke for or against research, whether they mentioned women or not, men consistently based their evaluations of embryo research and its technologies upon their assessment of the consequences for embryos or for the children that those embryos might become. Although women occasionally appeared within this 'discourse of the embryo', their role was subordinate to that of their potential or actual offspring. Women featured in men's arguments, not as primary agents, but as the bodies on which unborn children depend, as would-be mothers frustrated by their infertility, as grateful recipients of the benefits of science, as carers for the disabled, and as a convenient weapon with which to attack embryo research. In other words, when men were speaking, women were treated as marginal to the fundamental issues of the debate.

A rhetoric of women's experience

At the end of the final parliamentary debates on embryo research, men voted in favour of such research by a ratio of 2.2 to 1; women voted in favour by a ratio of 2.6 to 1. These figures show that female parliamentarians were, on the whole, slightly more likely than their male colleagues to support embryo research. There were significant variations, however, between women in the Upper and Lower Houses and within the two main political parties. In the Lords, although most women supported embryo research, they were less likely than men to vote in its favour.[20] In the Commons, in contrast, women were much more likely than men to vote for the continuation of research on human embryos. The dominance of pro-research views in the Lower House was due to the fact that the Labour Party had more female representatives there than did the Conservative Party. Conservative women in the Commons were actually more likely to vote against embryo research than to vote for it. But they were outnumbered and outvoted by women from the Labour Party and from the Liberal and Social Democratic Parties who were unanimously in favour of embryo research. In the final ballot in the House of Commons, nineteen Labour women plus six Conservatives and two women from the Liberal–Social Democratic Alliance voted for embryo research, whilst nine Conservative women voted against.

During the final phase of parliamentary debate, female representatives were divided into two distinct groupings whose members differed, not only in their votes and in their judgments concerning the legitimacy of embryo research, but also in their moral perspectives and their use of language. On the one hand, there was a minority group opposed to such research which drew its membership in both Houses predominantly from the Conservative Party. On the other hand, there was a larger group of women strongly in favour of embryo research drawn mainly from the Labour Party. The contributions of the former group of women to the parliamentary debate were similar to those of men opposed to embryo research. The arguments employed by these women were largely derived from the anti-abortion movement and, like the great majority of men, they insisted that the proper treatment of the human embryo was the central issue of the debate.[21] The members of the second group of women adopted a distinctive approach to the evaluation of embryo research which differed, not only from that of their male and female opponents, but also from that used by the male supporters of embryo research. Unlike all other groups, these women tried consistently to place women, rather than embryos, at the centre of the debate. They based their support for such research on the claim advanced in the opening debates that women had a special understanding of matters relating to reproduction and on the proposal that women's experiences of childbirth and pregnancy clearly demonstrated that research on human embryos should be allowed to continue.

Given that so much of parliamentary debate was concerned with the nature of the human embryo, female supporters of embryo research were unable entirely to ignore this issue. Frequently, however, when they dealt with this topic, they reversed the logic of the analysis adopted by men and by female critics of embryo research.

It is only when a woman misses her period that she suspects that she might be pregnant. Research that may assist infertile couples or women who frequently miscarry,
or which may identify hereditary defects, is undertaken during the period when the
fertilized egg may or may not become an embryo, then a fetus, and finally a baby.[22]

By no means will every fertilized egg result in a baby. A fertilized egg may try to
develop in the tubes and may never reach the womb. Its relationship to the mother
is one of a malignant growth that will kill her if allowed to develop. So how can I
agree with hon. Members who want me to regard such an entity as a human being?[23]

Female advocates of embryo research seldom attempted to establish the
status of the isolated human embryo and then to infer how such a being
should be treated. Rather, as in these two quotations, they assumed the
primacy of women's experience, such as the experience of the menstrual
cycle or of ectopic pregnancy, and from this they derived their view of the
embryo and of its rights.

In order to give voice to women's experiences, such speakers tended to
employ a distinctive linguistic style. In particular, they regularly built their
arguments around accounts of concrete, personal occurrences instead of
using the more generalized, impersonal argumentation about biological
processes or moral values on which men tended to rely. Female supporters
of embryo research repeatedly spoke about their own, and other women's,
direct involvement in pregnancy and childbirth. Although some male and
female critics of embryo research drew on personal experience of the effects
of genetic disorders within their own family, they were unable to match the
dramatic personal narratives provided by the women who supported
embryo research.[24] The following, heavily edited, quotation furnishes some
illustration of this style:

I shall make one personal point, as I am one of the few people in the Chamber who
has had an amniocentesis test when I had a child at the age of 39 . . . it took a further
seven weeks for the results of the blood test to be made available to my consultant,
who then agreed that I had had rubella at 13 weeks' pregnancy. I had spent seven
weeks knowing that the child was growing, becoming more obviously pregnant and
feeling it move. I was then given 24 hours to decide whether I wanted a termination.
I shall never forget those 24 hours in my life. I went ahead with the pregnancy and
my son . . . has been a great joy to us.[25]

Personal accounts of this kind were repeatedly used to draw attention to the
sorts of difficulties that could be faced by any woman. Those speakers who
had been spared such experiences often commented on their own good
fortune. At the same time, these exemplary stories were used to suggest how
such problems might eventually be overcome by the introduction of new,
science-based techniques. Thus, the speaker in the preceding passage

brought her account to a close by urging her audience to consider the wider implications of her particular experience:

I must stress to those who have never had the experience that that seven-week period was a miserable time and that the decision whether to go ahead with the pregnancy, knowing that I might have a severely disabled child or whether to abort a child who was quite well and would have a reasonable chance of happiness and fulfilment, was a dreadful one, and I would not wish it on anyone. It would be a great step forward for humanity for anyone to be able to make that decision in advance of having a child growing in their womb, and we should not turn our back on that option.[26]

By the end of this passage, the woman is no longer telling her own story, but is speaking on behalf of anyone who has had, or could have, a 'child growing in their womb'. In other words, the voice has become that of women in general speaking in favour of the new technologies as solutions to their reproductive problems. This speaker's adoption of the generic woman's voice is accomplished implicitly in the course of her extended narrative. Other female speakers made it clear from the start that they were speaking *as* a woman *on behalf* of women.[27] Men frequently claimed to speak as lawyers, as clergymen, as scientists, but never as a man representing men's interests. Female speakers arguing for embryo research, however, regularly identified themselves as women and put forward views which they presented as growing out of women's collective experience. In men's speeches, there was little awareness of the possibility of there being systematic differences of perspective between women and men in relation to the issues under discussion. In contrast, a number of female supporters of embryo research drew attention to men's persistent failure to appreciate 'the woman's point of view'.

100 years ago . . . hon. Gentlemen in this House were telling Queen Victoria that they positively knew that God was against the use of painkillers when giving birth – advice that she rightly rejected. But other women at that time could have taken that advice and refused painkillers when giving birth. Such refusal now would be supported by only a tiny minority.[28]

It makes me smile when I hear contraception talked about in this House as though it is entirely a Third World issue . . . I remind hon. Members that there are women in this country as well. The battle for a safe, effective, convenient form of contraception is still far from won.[29]

Some hon. Members may have seen a placenta. It is certainly human tissue and it is certainly useful. However, there would be considerable debate as to whether it had a human soul.[30]

In passages such as these, we can observe female speakers trying to convey to the male majority that women's understandings and preferences, which should have been central to the debate, had not been given their due consideration. In each of these quotations, there is at least a hint of derision; a suggestion that men's talk about childbirth, birth control and embryos is often hypocritical and divorced from the reality to be found in women's first-hand experience. This is most strikingly expressed by the last speaker who seems to imply that most of the serried ranks of men by whom she is surrounded had never come within touching distance of a placenta and that, for this reason alone, their abstract arguments concerning the ethical status of the embryo were suspect, if not entirely irrelevant.

The case made by those women who supported embryo research was essentially that many women encountered problems in the course of reproduction and that research involving human embryos gave women hope that some of these problems might be eliminated or, at least, made less severe. They often mentioned that they had visited an IVF clinic or a research establishment in order to ascertain how women undergoing treatment thought about these issues. Such visits were always cited as providing evidence in favour of research. The low success rates of IVF were seen, not as a sign of failure, but as indicating the need for further research. No mention was made of complaints from women receiving treatment at IVF centres or from women involved in research on assisted reproduction. There was not the least suggestion that women had been used in ways that they, or the speakers, found to be unacceptable. To the contrary, even those women who had not themselves benefited from the use of IVF were reported as wanting research and treatment to continue for the sake of others. The following quotation is typical:

> IVF has seemed almost like a miracle for desperately unhappy, childless couples who are able to undertake the new process . . . I have been able to visit the IVF clinic at Addenbrookes Hospital . . . I saw one woman who . . . had had the experience of delivering babies day by day while unable to have one of her own. She has had two failed IVF pregnancies but is now in the 25th week of her third pregnancy and is expecting twins . . . She understood the whole process and told me how strictly controlled the procedures are. What particularly delighted her was that almost all the patients . . . want to give their eggs for research because they want other women to have the chance that they have had, even if they themselves are not successful.[31]

During the final phase of parliamentary debate, female supporters of embryo research repeatedly drew attention to the feelings of women outside Parliament concerning assisted reproduction and research involving human embryos. They condemned their male colleagues for being insensitive to women's needs and they urged these men to listen more closely to women's testimony. They also provided detailed accounts of their own and of other women's reproductive experiences. These personal narratives were used time and again to support the claim that the great majority of women, and especially those with reproductive problems, approved unreservedly of embryo research and wanted it to continue.

Embryo research and happy families

It is clear from the parliamentary record that the female supporters of embryo research did not, in fact, speak for all women with direct experience of assisted reproduction. There were women outside Parliament who had used the new reproductive technology, but who were highly critical of its techniques and of the research with which it was associated. There was only one speech, however, in which women's negative experiences with assisted reproduction and embryo research were taken as the basis for an extended argument against the continuation of such research. The speaker was Baroness Elles in the last full debate in the Lords. Lady Elles spoke as follows:

I have had many letters and I have been approached by individuals and organizations, to ask in all this what the position of the woman is. It is the woman who has to produce the ova over the years to provide the necessary gametes which form the human embryo. We know there are shortages of eggs for research. We know that on sterilization women are asked to donate their eggs. What unconscious pressure will be put on women, for instance, to have sterilization? A woman said to me only yesterday that, IVF treatment having failed, she was left in a terrible situation. She is just one of the many of the 92 per cent who were given hormones and drug treatment with effects which are still not known . . . These women feel, rightly or wrongly, that they are being exploited by the scientists for the use of their eggs for human embryo research and for the use of drugs on their bodies in order to produce superovulation . . . Therefore, it should be said that if your Lordships, as men, had to undergo the forms of treatment under these new reproductive techniques . . . the vast majority would go into the Lobby voting against research.[32]

All the constituents are present in this speech for an anti-research rhetoric based on women's experiences with which to counter the pro-research rhetoric employed by the women who supported embryo research. But this potential counter-rhetoric was never adopted by other women in either House. Indeed, Lady Elles herself made a point of distancing herself from the claims of the women outside Parliament on whose behalf she was speaking. 'I use the words of these women,' she pointed out, 'they are not mine.'[33] Furthermore, her Ladyship's pleas were summarily dismissed by their Lordships. Lord Zuckerman, an eminent biologist, immediately insisted that the Baroness's argument raised no issue worthy of discussion in the House because the women in question must have gone voluntarily to the infertility clinics for help. The implication here seems to have been that these women would have given their informed consent to the treatment received at such clinics and, therefore, had no grounds for complaint. Lady Elles then asked if she might be allowed to reply. Hansard records that, at this juncture, various Noble Lords present in the Chamber shouted 'No!', and her Ladyship was forced to stay silent.[34] There followed a speech by Lord Jenkin in which he reasserted the customary view that those women who had experience of assisted reproduction were almost universally in favour of embryo research.[35] It appears that, at this late stage in the sequence of debates, the Members of the Upper House were unwilling to consider the possibility that many such women had not only not benefited from assisted reproduction, but might also have serious reservations about the continuation of embryo research.

Although Lady Elles's speech shows that there was a body of opinion antagonistic to embryo research among women with experience of assisted reproduction, this negative testimony was never given careful consideration in the course of parliamentary debate. It is possible that this critical view of embryo research was largely ignored by the women opposed to embryo research in Parliament because the latter either belonged to, or identified with, the anti-abortion movement; whilst the women with experience of the new reproductive technology would presumably have supported women's rights to control their own reproductive processes. In other words, it is possible that an anti-research rhetoric based on women's experience did not emerge in the course of parliamentary debate because those women in Parliament who rejected embryo research on principle and those women outside Parliament who condemned such research on the basis of personal experience were ideologically divided at a more basic level and, as a result, were unable to establish a shared moral framework.[36]

Whether or not this was the major reason, the female opponents of embryo research in Parliament seldom mentioned women's negative experiences of assisted reproduction. Consequently, virtually all the direct testimony that was cited from women outside Parliament during the closing debates expressed enthusiastic support for the continuation of embryo research. Thus, any parliamentarians who were receptive to the idea that women have a privileged understanding of the experiences and moral issues associated with assisted reproduction would almost certainly have been led towards support for embryo research by the evidence given concerning the experiences and preferences of ordinary women.

By the end of the long sequence of debate, parliamentary opinion finally settled with most Members of both sexes in close agreement about the legitimacy of research involving early human embryos. There was also general agreement about the benefits to be bestowed by such research on those who wished to enjoy ordinary family life. Women, in particular, repeatedly argued that they approved of embryo research and assisted reproduction because these developments would enable more people to enter more fully into the joys of domesticity. The support given to embryo research by women within Parliament was, like that of men, an expression of their commitment to the conventional family.

In a society which is built upon the family, people who are unable to have children feel shut out from life's most valuable experience, and their loneliness and frustration simply grows.[37]

There was a couple at the unit . . . It made one appreciate . . . how much the possibility of having a child meant to them. It would be dreadful if they did not have that opportunity . . . I hope that as a result of its provisions for research and treatment, in future many more couples will have the opportunity of producing healthy and much wanted babies.[38]

The opponents of embryo research, both men and women, refused to accept this positive vision of the future. They chose to regard such research as a serious long-term threat to the morality of family life. In their view research on human embryos, and the technologies to which it would give rise, were likely in due course to destroy the family they knew and valued. In contrast, the numerically dominant supporters of embryo research, both women and men, were confident that IVF and related techniques had already improved the quality of life for many families and that the scientific advances yet to come would continue this process.

The major parliamentary division, during the concluding debates, was not between women and men, but between opponents and supporters of embryo research. Most women belonged to the latter party; but so did most men. Amongst these supporters there was essential agreement that the new technologies of reproduction were compatible with normal family life and that it would not be difficult to ensure that they were used in ways that maintained the existing pattern of family relationships. Men's approach to these issues tended to begin with the interests of embryos and children, whilst that of women was more likely to begin with women's experiences. But these different points of departure were reconciled in a shared advocacy of family life where, it was assumed, the interests of embryos, children, mothers and fathers naturally converged.

7

Science and religion

Throughout the 1980s, the various Christian denominations in Britain drew upon their established systems of belief and moral principle to try to assess the legitimacy of embryo research and to offer guidance on this topic to their members. For example, in 1982, the Board of Social Responsibility of the Church of England set up a working party on human fertilization and embryology in order to 'apply Biblical understanding and Christian ethical tradition' to the issues arising from IVF and embryo research.[1] Similarly, the Roman Catholic Church looked closely at embryo research during this period and issued a series of formal judgments.[2] Although there was considerable resistance to embryo research on religious grounds, and in some quarters emphatic insistence that such research should be forbidden, the position adopted by the churches and by their members was by no means uniform and by no means consistently negative. For instance, the Archbishop of York, Primate of England, argued repeatedly on behalf of embryo research in Parliament and elsewhere.[3] Nevertheless, despite the diversity of religious opinion, some of those in favour of research on human embryos chose to depict the public debate over the rights and wrongs of embryo research as essentially a struggle between scientific rationality and religious dogma.

This view of the debate is clearly evident in the various references by supporters of embryo research to the scientific martyrdom of Galileo at the hands of religious extremists. Galileo was used by advocates of embryo research as a symbol of religious intolerance and as a warning against allowing the future of research on human embryos to be decided on the basis of religious considerations. The examples provided below have been taken from speeches made by Lady Warnock and by Lord Hailsham in the House of Lords. In such passages, speakers attempt to undermine their opponents by representing the debate over embryo research as a conflict between those who wish to enforce unthinking obedience to out-of-date religious beliefs and those who are determined to defend scientists' right to continue their search for the truth.[4]

In my view it would be in the last degree paradoxical if we, a democratic and an increasingly educated people, should, by rejecting [embryo research] put ourselves back into the seventeenth century when the question of whether or not Galileo and indeed Descartes might pursue and publish their scientific findings was regulated not by scientific but by religious considerations.[5]

Total prohibition [of embryo research] would involve going down a road which has failed every time it has been tried in history. It started before the time of Galileo and it was a road which led ultimately to Tyndale being strangled in a Dutch prison for translating the scriptures. It was the road which led Galileo to be condemned by the Holy Office. It is the road which ultimately has always failed.[6]

Galileo was an important point of reference within pro-research rhetoric, not only in Parliament, but also in other settings. For instance, a contributor to *New Scientist* in January 1990 was led to complain bitterly that 'a number of your correspondents appear to regard the embryo research debate as a re-run of Galileo-versus-the-Church . . . As an atheist, a trained scientist and a supporter of the pro-life movement I would strongly challenge this . . . It seems that some people would like to have their cake and eat it, accusing their opponents of religious fundamentalism, while themselves relying on woolly metaphysical arguments with little rational basis.'[7] As we can see from this response, the portrayal of the debate over embryo research as yet another clash between scientific rationality and religious dogma did not go uncontested. In the present chapter, I shall examine the adequacy of this 'Galilean' interpretation of the embryo debate in the parliamentary context. I shall concentrate on debate within the House of Lords[8] which, unlike the Commons, includes speakers drawn from the world of science as well as from the Church of England and from some of the other major religious communities to be found in present-day Britain.[9] I shall argue that the forms of argumentation linked to religion and science in the parliamentary forum cannot be distinguished in terms of their rationality, their reliance on dogma or in terms of other features central to the stereotyped contrast between religious and scientific styles of thought.[10] I shall also argue, however, that there were other, genuine, differences between the religious and the science-based contributions to the debate which help us to understand why the supporters of embryo research succeeded in overcoming the vigorous denunciations based on religion with which parliamentary debate began.

The contrast between reason and belief

In the initial debate on the Warnock Report in the House of Lords in 1984, the great majority of speakers condemned research involving human embryos on the grounds that the experimental use of living human organisms was morally repugnant and contrary to Christian principle. In the course of this debate, the speech most frequently cited with approval was that by the Marquess of Reading, who argued as follows:[11]

The whole of British law has been traditionally influenced by the Christian religion. That faith upholds the sanctity of every single human life. The principle of the sanctity of life may be perceived by reason alone. It is the cornerstone of the natural law, without which all morality would be a matter of opinion. The principle is also upheld in the Christian faith . . . Clearly the Old Testament . . . ascribes personhood to the developing embryo without benefit of the contemporary scientific knowledge of the individuality of the fetus. The embryo is referred to in personal terms rather than as a bundle of protoplasm and blood. This is taken a step further in the New Testament . . . Therefore, in conclusion, human life, created in the image and likeness of God, has intrinsic value irrespective of its maturity or the development of functional skills. Thus embryonic human beings are the same person that they will be when they are older and more developed . . . To create, in the laboratory, isolated human beings for the purpose of experimentation, or to use so-called 'spare' embryos for that purpose, represents a blatant disregard for the civil rights of those human beings, as well as endorsing the principle that we can be justified in defining some human persons as non-persons in order to use them for our own interests.[12]

The two basic components of this argument are advocacy of the principle of the sanctity of each individual human life, and the assertion that the early human embryo is a living person. These elements together generate the conclusion that research on early human embryos is immoral and should not be allowed in a Christian, or indeed in any civilized, society.

Embryo research was condemned in this fashion, not only by those speaking explicitly as members of a religious faith, but also by those who claimed no specific religious identity. The Marquess of Reading implied that the exercise of moral reasoning, even without religious guidance, would lead naturally to this conclusion, and several speakers suggested that repudiation of research on living human embryos was more or less universal. The Bishop of Norwich, for example, referred to a MORI poll showing that 85 per cent of people in Britain 'felt that experiments on human embryos were not right'.[13] The Marquess of Lothian maintained that the sanctity of the human embryo and the immorality of embryo research was 'something with which practically all religious denominations and faiths in the world would assent'.[14] Thus, unequivocal rejection of embryo research on moral and religious grounds was the dominant reaction in the first debate on this topic in the House of Lords. This response was portrayed as an expression of a broad moral consensus present in society at large.[15]

The next debate on embryo research in the Lords occurred early in 1988, after a delay of slightly more than two years. By this time, those in favour of embryo research had become much more organized and better prepared to engage in parliamentary confrontation. As a result, on this occasion, twelve of the twenty-one contributors spoke for embryo research, while only seven spoke against.[16] In the opening debate, the few supporters of embryo research had been defensive and apologetic.[17] In the second debate, however, the advocates of embryo research were much more aggressive and sought to build a case for such research, not only by presenting positive arguments in its favour, but also by attacking the credibility of their opponents. This was done, in part, by adopting the 'Galilean' view of opposition to embryo research, and by presenting an invidious comparison between their own detached assessment of the evidence and their adversaries' dogmatic reliance on religious authority. This tactic can be seen at work in the following passage in which Lord Henderson, one of the leading supporters of embryo research, launches an attack upon the Duke of Norfolk, who had earlier rejected such research on religious and moral grounds:

> The Duke of Norfolk . . . was the first speaker . . . who used the important words 'I believe'. Others had not rested their arguments on belief. The noble Duke, with characteristic forthrightness and honesty, used the words 'I believe' at the outset of his speech. Again . . . he said that he was following the Catholic line. I very much respect that. They were key words in his speech, and perhaps in the speeches of other Catholics and Christians who particularly brought their belief before the House. It is a case of not being able to argue with belief. One never can. The noble Baroness, Lady Warnock, most eloquently said so in her speech . . . I do not propose to argue with what the noble Duke said. I respect his remarks but I shall leave them on one side because it is not an arguable matter . . . the Duke of Norfolk expressly based his arguments on belief and authority.[18]

There are no Roman Catholic clergy in the House of Lords. It therefore falls to the Catholic nobility, first among whom is the Duke of Norfolk,[19] to represent the Catholic viewpoint on moral issues in the Upper House. In placing special emphasis on the Duke's opposition to embryo research, Lord Henderson was attacking Catholic resistance to such research, in particular, as well as the position taken by those other Christians who had decided that embryo research was immoral. His Lordship's central accusation was that opposition by Catholics and by other Christians originated largely from unthinking acceptance of religious belief and from uncritical compliance with clerical authority.

From this interpretation of religious opposition to embryo research, Lord Henderson inferred that there was no point in trying to argue rationally with his opponents because their opinions on this topic were rigid and unchangeable. His Lordship did not state explicitly what he would have recommended in place of belief and authority. It was evident elsewhere in his speech, however, that he regarded his own position on embryo research as a reasoned response to the scientific facts about human embryos. Furthermore, the view that belief/faith and authority should be replaced by reason and fact had already been presented forcefully in the speech by Lady Warnock which Lord Henderson cited with warm approval:

Those who argue that research using human embryos should become a criminal offence . . . do so on the grounds . . . that it is already an offence to use children or non-consenting adults for medical research, and that the law should afford the same protection to embryos and fetuses from the moment of fertilization. They hold that the life of an individual begins at fertilization and that it is immaterial, after fertilization, whether that individual has or has not been born. I honour the sincerity and loyalty of those who adhere to that principle. However, it must be emphasized that the principle is founded on faith and not upon reason or the demonstration of facts. Arguments will not prove relevant to the principle because no demonstration of the great goods that will flow from the research . . . could be expected to move those who, as a matter of faith, hold that all human life is, or should be, equally protected by law from the moment of fertilization . . . It is to human individuals that our duty and our care must belong morally. But it is factually impossible . . . to think of the pre-embryo as an individual with an individual life to lead.[20]

Lady Warnock and Lord Henderson led the counter-attack on behalf of embryo research against its religious opponents. In their attempts to undermine this opposition, they employed the familiar, stereotyped contrast between religious thinking and thinking that adopts a more scientific approach.[21] The former was said to depend ultimately on faith or belief; the latter on reason. The former was said to involve the uncritical repetition of fixed dogma; the latter to follow from open-minded appraisal. The former was said to rely on authoritative pronouncement; the latter on demonstration of the facts. This 'Galilean' interpretation of the contest over embryo research entered formal parliamentary debate during the session in 1988 in which the initial ascendancy of the religious opponents of such research was first seriously challenged. Thereafter, the stereotyped contrast between science and religion was used on a regular basis by the leading supporters of embryo research.[22]

Similarities in moral reasoning

The denunciation of 'woolly-minded' religious thinking by the pro-research lobby was intended to persuade those who were undecided about embryo research to give less credence to the claims of its opponents.[23] Although it is unlikely that this kind of generalized condemnation of religious opposition had a decisive impact on the outcome of the parliamentary process, some of those who continued to resist embryo research on religious grounds regarded these accusations of religious absolutism as sufficiently serious to require rebuttal. They responded to the attack by insisting that, although their rejection of such research was unequivocal, it was nevertheless a considered view, based on reason and respect for evidence. The following example is taken from the next debate in the parliamentary series:[24]

Speakers on the last occasion said that the contest was between reason, which they saw themselves representing, and faith – presumably it was some muddled, irrational form of faith which they attributed to the Christian lobby. I am afraid I do not accept that way of looking at the issue. All this work has been done by these theologians, doctors and scientists and they have reached certain conclusions which put them at least equal with any scientist that the noble Baroness, Lady Warnock, has been able to mobilize . . . I do not think we can say that on the one side there is reason and scientific research and on the other a lot of hot gospellers or Roman acolytes . . . I would never stand up and support [these views] if I had not reached that conclusion and if I did not in conscience consider that these were reasonable views. There are other views held with deep sincerity. I appreciate that but let us not talk as though reason was on one side and faith on the other, even, as it is often implied, a rather idiotic faith. There is reason on both sides.[25]

In this passage, Lord Longford tried to redress the imbalance built into the stereotyped contrast between science and religion in relation to embryo research. He did not denounce his opponents, in turn, as unreasonable, but sought to re-establish, more tolerantly, that there was reason on both sides. His Lordship could have developed his defence of religious thinking further by pointing out that the basic structure of moral argument was identical on both sides of the debate in that they both endorsed the principle of the sanctity of human life and both regarded research on human individuals as immoral. The critical difference between the two sides lay, not in their overall style or structure of argumentation, but in their judgment of when the developing human embryo becomes an individual and, accordingly, when the moral principle requiring protection of the individual comes into effect. Those opposed to embryo research argued that human individuals come into being with the genetic union brought about by the merging of sperm and egg. Given the principle of the sanctity of human life, it seemed to follow logically that human embryos should be protected from the time of fertilization, and that all research on such embryos should be forbidden. Those in favour of research argued that human individuals do not start to emerge until certain structural developments have occurred in the embryo about two weeks after fertilization. Given the principle of the sanctity of human life, it seemed to follow logically from this alternative view of the embryo that research on embryos that are more than two weeks from fertilization should be forbidden, but that research is permissible on the pre-fourteen-day embryo or 'pre-embryo'.[26]

The two sides in the debate over embryo research were in agreement about the limits that applied to scientific research involving adults, children, fetuses and post-fourteen-day embryos.[27] They differed only over the nature, moral standing and proper treatment of the very early human embryo. Lady Warnock, Lord Henderson and their supporters made no attempt to explain why the Christian opponents of embryo research suddenly became infected with moral irrationality when dealing with the early embryo, even though the rest of their moral reasoning appeared to be unblemished.[28] Nor did the defenders of embryo research say how they were able to recognize the supposed absence of reason and the supposed disrespect for scientific evidence within the 'Christian lobby', apart from the fact that its members reached conclusions different from theirs about the legitimacy of research on early human embryos. Furthermore, those who *supported* embryo research on religious grounds were never accused of irrationality. In other words, no independent evidence of the distorting impact of religious belief was required. Departure from the procedures of reasoned thought was simply taken to be self-evident in those cases where opponents of embryo research openly acknowledged their religious commitments and were also unwilling to support this area of scientific inquiry.[29]

Lord Henderson complained on behalf of the pro-research lobby that 'one simply cannot argue with these Catholics and other Christians who simply bring their dogmatic beliefs about the human embryo before the House'.[30] However, when Lord Henderson said 'one cannot argue with these people', he meant, in effect, that he could not persuade them to agree with *him*. Similarly, when Lady Warnock observed that 'arguments will not prove relevant' to her adversaries, she was referring only to those arguments that *she* found convincing but which were unacceptable to those who did not share her view of the early human embryo.[31]

This contemptuous dismissal of Christian opposition to embryo research by Lady Warnock, Lord Henderson and other leading figures in favour of such research[32] can itself be seen as dogmatic and as dependent on authoritative pronouncement. For example, in the passage quoted above, we have observed Lady Warnock insisting that it was 'factually impossible to think of the pre-embryo as an individual with an individual life to lead'.[33] This statement seems to suggest that anyone who disagreed with her about the emergence of the human individual at day fourteen was either choosing to ignore relevant facts or was imposing interpretations upon them which were obviously untenable. In many speeches, however, the opponents of embryo research appear to have been as committed as Lady Warnock and her supporters to careful assessment of the evidence.

Let me come to the heart of the matter which is this. Before conception there are two conglomerations of cells called a sperm and an ovum, neither of which, if given the best treatment . . . will turn into human beings. Immediately after conception, there is something I should like to call a 'conceptus' . . . The 'conceptus', if given the best treatment, will turn into a human being . . . It is obviously not possible to assimilate the 'conceptus' to anything that has gone before . . . and it is very easy to assimilate it to what comes after . . . Indeed, it contains that bundle of cells which the pro-research faction want to call the embryo. There is an unbroken time progression and an unbroken ontological process from the moment of conception to the moment of death.[34]

It is, of course, perfectly reasonable to disagree with this conclusion on the grounds that a small proportion of early embryos become twins or that the first signs of internal organization do not appear until two weeks after conception. But Lady Warnock's rejection of her opponents' arguments as 'factually impossible' seems to convey an unwillingness to consider seriously any alternative interpretation of the facts about early embryos or to recognize the possible validity of any moral stance which differs from her own. The tendentious nature of her position becomes evident when we note the statement in the Warnock Report that questions concerning the origin of individual human beings can never be decided solely by reference to the factual realm: 'Although the questions of when life or personhood begin appear to be questions of fact susceptible of straightforward answers, we hold that the answers to such questions in fact are complex amalgams of factual and moral judgments.'[35]

In the course of public debate over embryo research, Lady Warnock and her colleagues in the House of Lords appear to have abandoned this view, which might have allowed both sides legitimately to reach different conclusions, and to have insisted instead that the scientific facts about the early human embryo unambiguously resolved the moral issues under discussion. Ironically, in denouncing as dogmatism their opponents' refusal to accept these supposed facts, the leading advocates of embryo research came to present their own claims in a manner that allowed no room for reconsideration or compromise. This can be seen clearly in Lord Henderson's account of why he regarded scientific experiment involving pre-fourteen-day embryos to be acceptable:

In no sense can the 14-day period be regarded as an embryo. That has been made clear by today's speeches. It has been made very clear by the experts to whom I have listened over the years. I instance particularly . . . Dr Winston . . . Dr McLaren and Prof. Shaw . . . These humane people made the distinction so clear to me that I find that the moral problem of dealing with the first 14 days after fertilization of the embryo has disappeared . . . As a result of the absolute certainty this medical opinion has given me, I find that there is no moral problem.[36]

In this passage, we find Lord Henderson claiming 'absolute certainty' for his current, 'scientific', view of the embryo, and hence for his current moral position. Although he was never given the chance, it would have been entirely appropriate in the circumstances if the Duke of Norfolk had adopted his opponent's vocabulary and replied with the words: 'I respect his remarks but I shall leave them on one side because it is not an arguable matter.'[37] Both Lord Henderson, with his 'absolute certainty', and Lady Warnock, with her 'factual impossibility', seem open to the charge of 'factual absolutism'; that is, of being unwilling in principle to consider any arguments incompatible with their present understanding of the facts. Furthermore, as the last quotation shows, the lay supporters of embryo research were entirely dependent upon the experts engaged in embryo research for their 'facts' concerning the early human embryo. Thus, like those participants who 'followed the Catholic line', many pro-researchers justified their own position by means of pronouncements about the embryo which they took to be unarguable, and which originated from external sources that they deemed to be authoritative.[38]

The lay supporters of embryo research in the Lords were heavily dependent on the scientific community for their arguments and, in particular, for their view of the early embryo. Once they had accepted the scientists' case, however, lay supporters tended to treat the scientists' claims as unmediated representations of the nature of things. They came to regard their science-based 'facts' as different in kind from the 'traditional beliefs' or the 'untested edicts' cited by the religious authorities.[39] In other words, it was assumed by many lay supporters of embryo research that the authority of science was superior to that of other sources; and that science could be used to resolve the moral issues arising from such research with a degree of certainty not otherwise available.[40]

Given this assumption, we might have expected those eminent scientists who participated in the debate to have reaffirmed the special authority of science and to have stressed the importance of scientific testimony. Yet, when we consider the parliamentary speeches made by the representatives of the scientific community, we find that their assessment of the role of scientific evidence in the debate was much more restrained than that of their more enthusiastic supporters. Scientists did argue fairly consistently in favour of embryo research and they did claim to know many facts about human embryos. But scientists themselves never maintained that these facts could be used unequivocally to decide the moral issues under examination; nor did they endorse the suggestion that those arguing the case for embryo research had special access to the realm of rational thought.[41]

Finally, I should say that I recognize that a moral judgment underlies this debate. From that point of view my opinion as a scientist probably has no greater value than that of any layman who has bent his thoughts to the matters we are discussing. I fully recognize that there are limits to the rational exercise of scientific method, not only as regards intellectual inquiry but also very much more so in the determination of moral issues. Science will never provide the answers to the ultimate questions: the question of what brought about what we call life and what it is that gives man his unique quality in the world of living organisms.[42]

In summary, when we survey the series of parliamentary debates over embryo research, we can see that the 'Galilean' contrast between science and religion became prominent in the contributions of those lay speakers who led the counter-attack on the 'Christian lobby' during the debates in 1988–9. The basic assertion made by these speakers – that the two sides in the debate were divided, not only by different views of embryo research, but also by fundamentally different styles of argumentation – was unfounded. This claim was no more than a rhetorical restatement of differences of opinion concerning the nature of the early human embryo dressed up in terms of the stereotyped contrast between religious and scientific styles of thought. In practice, both sides in the debate made use of scientific 'facts' in justifying their moral stance;[43] both sides interpreted these facts 'reasonably' in the light of broad moral principle; both sides relied on the judgments of 'experts'; and both sides were capable of presenting their case in a 'dogmatic' manner. The basic moral principle of the sanctity of human life was shared by all contributors to the debate, and its application to scientific research was agreed in all areas except that of the early human embryo. Rather than being divided by contrary styles of thought, the two sides were bound together by a common religious and moral tradition and by a common respect for evidence and for reasoned argument.

Nevertheless, despite these similarities, the two sides were unable to agree. Despite their common cultural inheritance, they found themselves engaged in a prolonged, and sometimes bitter, confrontation which ended, not in consensus, but in resort to the ballot box. In the next section, I shall look more closely at what actually separated the two sides and at how these differences led to the parliamentary victory of those who claimed to speak on behalf of science.

Religious disunity and scientific consensus

In the opening debate on embryo research in the Lords, one speaker after another stood up to condemn such research as morally offensive. Within a few weeks, a similar wave of moral revulsion swept through the Commons. This negative reaction to experimentation on human embryos was said to be part of a wider tide of moral disapproval which was almost universal within society at large, and which followed naturally from the application of generally accepted Christian principles. Yet, even at this stage, when parliamentary opposition to embryo research was at its height, there were still a few parliamentarians who insisted that research of this kind was not incompatible with Christian belief. As the sequence of discussions continued, this minority view became more widespread, and the early claims concerning the existence of a moral and religious consensus in opposition to embryo research became less frequent and less credible as the divisions within religious opinion became increasingly evident. In due course, the lack of religious unity with respect to embryo research came to be openly acknowledged, even by those most firmly opposed to such research on religious grounds.[44]

One reason for the absence of a unified and lasting response to embryo research based on religion is that Christianity, the dominant form of religion in the British Parliament, is itself divided into numerous different traditions.[45] Each separate tradition, in turn, contains many potentially discrepant cultural elements which can be used to justify quite different evaluations of modern science and technology. The following passage provides a brief summary of some of the conflicting strands of belief that are present within the major Christian denominations and that are likely to be brought to bear, in various different ways, in attempts to assess new scientific developments such as those associated with embryo research.

First, the Bible holds up a distinctive view of *human fulfilment*. It does not minimize the importance of food and shelter and health . . . there are repeated calls for action to alleviate physical suffering . . . Much of modern technology, especially in agriculture and medicine, can be seen as a response to such physical needs . . . [However, fulfilment also] consists of right relationship to God and neighbour . . . Respect for human dignity today includes sensitivity to the effects of technology on people and

the subtle ways in which persons can be manipulated . . . Receptivity and acknowl-
edgment of grace stand in contrast to the attitudes of control and manipulation
which a technological society encourages. The Christian tradition cherishes dimensions of human experience which are not accessible to technical reason.

Second, the biblical view of *human nature* combines realism with idealism . . . The
recognition of human fallibility and the abuse of power should make us hesitant to
turn over social decisions to technical experts, however well-intentioned . . . But the
biblical tradition is also idealistic in its vision of creative human potentialities and
the possibility of a more just social order.[46]

The sacred texts of Christianity can easily generate both favourable and
unfavourable interpretations of advances in science and technology.
Improvements in technical control, such as control over the biological
processes of human reproduction, can be taken to be steps towards greater
fulfilment of human need and the establishment of a more Christian
society; but they may also be seen to involve improper manipulation of
human individuals and to lead towards a dangerous lessening of respect for
human dignity. In the case of embryo research, the balance between these
opposing evaluative tendencies depended critically on participants' judgments concerning the nature of the early human embryo. In the first stage
of parliamentary debate, as we have seen, most contributors agreed that
there was clear biblical warrant for regarding the early human embryo as a
person with full moral status; and, therefore, for concluding that experimental manipulation of human embryos was immoral. As the debate proceeded, however, many Christians found themselves unable to sustain this
reading of biblical sources.

Christians have a rather difficult time because it is no good looking in the New
Testament – I speak subject to the guidance of two Bishops – because we shall not
find in it what our Lord said about embryos. It is a question of the development of
Christian doctrine, and undoubtedly there is more than one view taken in the
Church as a whole.[47]

As a Christian I find this issue one of the most difficult I have ever had to wrestle
with. Initially I felt inclined to agree with the minority view of the Warnock Report
– that we should not have any research – because I believe that research could very
easily get out of control and lead to real damage, and in itself it is repugnant to do
research on anything approaching a human being, even a potential human being
. . . I am no expert but I have visited one of the medical research units doing this
work . . . As I understand it and as experts have told me – several have confirmed
it – there is an element of instability in the embryo up to about [fourteen days]. I
therefore agree with [the Bishop of Ripon] that it is impossible to put forward the
view that an embryo which might become one individual or two individuals in the
future can in religious terms have a soul . . . I believe deeply that research should
not be banned.[48]

In the later stages of parliamentary debate, the appearance of religious unity was replaced by evaluative diversity and by confrontation over the morality of embryo research among those speaking as Christians. Whether they spoke for or against such research, Christians increasingly found themselves adopting an interpretation of the human embryo and an assessment of embryo research that was firmly rejected, not just by other Christians, but by other members of their own religious denomination. This was least true among the Roman Catholics who, on the whole, continued to endorse the formal condemnation of embryo research proclaimed by the Church authorities. But there was disagreement on this matter even among the Catholics.[49]

My wife and I are practising Roman Catholics . . . The argument against [embryo] research turns, as many speakers have said, on the exact time at which life begins. The point has also been made a number of times that Christian theological thought regarding ensoulment or animation has changed over the years. Until the last century the critical point in time was certainly taken to be much later than 14 days after fertilization. There is still a range of opinion among theologians and we have heard some of these opinions in the debate . . . Noble Lords have heard the arguments about twinning, the wastage of fertilized eggs and the individuation of cells. I do not propose to repeat them. I find them sufficiently persuasive to enable me at least to contemplate the possibility that the destruction of defective embryos, under strict statutory control and up to 14 days after fertilization, may not be intrinsically wrong.[50]

The internal division of religious opinion was most pronounced among the Anglicans, who constituted by far the largest religious grouping in the Lords. These parliamentary differences reflected the lack of agreement on this topic within the Church of England itself. For example, in the fifty-five pages of the report of the working party set up by the Church of England to provide guidance on matters related to embryo research and assisted reproduction, there were seventeen explicit references to disagreement among its members and only two references to agreement. The report concluded that there were irreconcilable differences of philosophical perspective with regard to the nature and development of human personhood within the Anglican community, as there were within society as a whole.[51] Consequently, the members of the working party were themselves unable to agree about the status of the early human embryo or to offer a firm judgment concerning the legitimacy of research involving such embryos.[52]

It is probable that these divisions were largely responsible for the marked reluctance among the Anglican bishops in the Lords to contribute to the series of debates over the important moral issues associated with research on human embryos. Thus, only seven of the one hundred and thirty-two speeches in the five major debates were delivered by Anglican bishops or archbishops; only five of the twenty-six bishops and archbishops with seats in the Lords actually took part in the debates; and only six of them voted on embryo research in February 1990, two voting for and four against its continuation. Those few members of the bench of bishops and archbishops who did participate actively in the parliamentary process in the later debates tended to emphasize the absence of a unified Anglican view.

The Board of Social Responsibility of the General Synod of the Church of England was, by a majority, in favour of research on human embryos up to 14 days. A minority opposed that view. However, the board was opposed to the direct production of embryos for the sole purpose of research. The General Synod of the Church of England has voted twice on the matter. Both votes indicated a fairly even division of opinion within the Synod. It is therefore clear that the Church does not speak with one voice on this matter.[53]

Those Anglican bishops who contributed to the later stages of parliamentary debate did not attempt to define the Christian, or even the Anglican, position on embryo research. They spoke rather, as the Archbishop of York put it, 'primarily in a personal capacity',[54] and tried to convey their own individual interpretation of how the scriptures and the Christian tradition might be used to approach the moral issues surrounding such research. The overall balance of Anglican clerical opinion in Parliament remained opposed to the continuation of experimentation involving human embryos. However, as a result of the marked differences among the Anglican clergy, along with the presence of varied opinions among the Catholics and other Christian denominations,[55] it became difficult for any speaker arguing from religious belief to maintain that there was either a distinctive Christian view of the early human embryo or a single Christian answer to the moral questions raised by embryo research.

As the lengthy parliamentary appraisal of embryo research took its course, religious opinion became increasingly divided. Although opposition to such research continued to have a strong religious component, the growing number of parliamentarians in favour of research also drew freely upon religious sources to justify their contrary position. The leading advocates of embryo research took advantage of this situation to try to discredit the arguments of their opponents.

I am not in the least opposed to any Christian teaching putting forward the views that it believes to be true with regard to the value of human life from the two-cell stage onwards. As we have heard, there is profound disagreement among Christians about this teaching. As I have said and as we have already heard, there are numbers of bishops and scientists who must be allowed to be Christian and who hold differing views from those we have heard expressed . . . In my view it would be morally wrong to place obstacles derived from beliefs that are not very widely shared in the path of science, and especially in the path of science and the practice of medicine.[56]

In this passage, Lady Warnock contrasts the 'profound disagreement among Christians' in relation to embryo research with the apparently unified view to be found within the scientific and medical communities. Although she does not make it fully explicit, she seems to assume that the practitioners of science and medicine differed from the interpreters of religious belief in being essentially in agreement about the legitimacy of embryo research and about the path that those involved in such research should be allowed to follow.

This implicit comparison between religious disunity and scientific consensus over embryo research was largely justified. There were, it is true, a few scientists who were publicly critical of research on human embryos and who expressed doubts about its necessity and/or its morality. The parliamentary critics of embryo research paid particular attention to the statements made by these individuals.[57] However, all the major sources of authoritative scientific opinion in the UK, such as the Royal Society, the Medical Research Council, the British Medical Association and the Royal Society of Obstetricians and Gynaecologists, pronounced emphatically in favour of such research.[58] At the same time, the scientific representatives in the House of Lords, unlike the bishops, participated actively in parliamentary debate; especially during the closing stages when Government legislation was about to be enacted. Thus, nine out of eighteen scientist-peers spoke in the major debates, contributing a total of sixteen speeches. In the crucial debate in December 1989, seven scientists took part, compared with one member of the bench of bishops. All these lords of science argued strongly in favour of embryo research and every scientific speaker voted for its continuation.[59] Unlike the bishops, the scientists spoke confidently on behalf of a unified community of technical experts in terms designed to allay people's anxieties about the experimental manipulation of human subjects and to convince them of the immense benefits that were potentially available.[60]

Opposition to embryo research depended heavily on reference to religious belief and to the sacred texts of Christianity. The arguments of those opposed to such research were seriously weakened by the progressive fragmentation of religious opinion. In contrast, the arguments of those who supported embryo research were strengthened by the public unity of scientific and medical opinion.[61] In the absence of clear religious guidance,[62] parliamentarians turned increasingly for help to the scientific community. The scientific experts, although they claimed no special competence in matters of morality, welcomed the parliamentary decision-makers into their clinics and laboratories and succeeded in convincing many of them, both Christians and others, that the early embryo is not a person, that there is no conflict between embryo research and Christian values, that the products of such research would be overwhelmingly beneficial and, therefore, that experimentation involving human embryos should be allowed to continue.

The concerted arguments presented by the scientific community, combined with the diversity of religious views, had a double effect on parliamentary opinion. In the first place, it made the initial condemnation of embryo research seem more and more doubtful. At the same time, it made the sacrifice of therapeutic benefits required by that condemnation appear more and more costly. The most important of the promised benefits of embryo research was the eventual control of many forms of genetic disease by means of selective screening of IVF embryos. As we have seen, Members of both Houses found this promise particularly persuasive. Clinical control over the transmission of genetic diseases had not actually been achieved at the time of these debates. Nevertheless, the firm anticipation of success in this field by practising scientists and by figures of scientific authority was enough to convince the majority of parliamentarians that further research on human embryos should go ahead.

The belief by lay persons that scientists would be able to deliver effective control over a wide range of genetic diseases in a form that would benefit the population at large was critical in establishing a substantial parliamentary majority in the Lords in favour of embryo research. Once this majority existed, it became possible for supporters of such research further to strengthen their case by reference to the basic democratic principle of the right of the majority to pursue their collective interests as long as their actions cause no harm to the minority.

No one can doubt that the overwhelming weight of scientific and medical opinion is in favour of such research . . . The legislator must master, at least in outline, the medical and scientific issues with which he has to deal. However, in a democratic, pluralist society he must also weigh conflicting opinions and be aware that those who oppose research are in a minority . . . Democratic legislators accept that the beliefs of minorities should, if possible, not be outraged by the majority. But they know too that minorities cannot be permitted to coerce the majority, the more especially in this instance because no member of the minority will be compelled by this Bill to use or benefit from the results of the research which the minority finds repugnant. For those reasons I trust that the House will support . . . the continuance of research on pre-embryos.[63]

During the last few months of parliamentary debate, this kind of reference to democratic principle occurred regularly in speeches on behalf of embryo research.[64] This new argument implicitly divided Parliament, and the wider society, into two distinct moral groupings. On the one hand, there was taken to be a minority whose members were dogmatically committed to a narrow interpretation of Christian values, who believed that embryo research was wrong and who insisted that its potential benefits were morally tainted. On the other hand, it was implied that there was a majority whose members had succeeded in responding constructively to the challenge posed by embryo research, who understood that such research was morally legitimate and who were keen to ensure that its therapeutic benefits were made quickly available. The proposed legislation, it was argued, allowed the former grouping to retain its beliefs and to refuse to take advantage of the forthcoming benefits, whilst enabling scientists to proceed with the restricted range of inquiries enthusiastically approved by the moral majority. In a modern, pluralist society, it was suggested, this tolerant recognition of the existence of distinct moral communities was the only realistic solution.

Dogma, authority and faith

The parliamentary debate over embryo research was often depicted as a confrontation between religious dogma and scientific rationality. I have argued that this interpretation of the struggle over embryo research may well have been a useful adversarial device, but that it does not provide an accurate description. I have tried to show that those opposed to embryo research and those in favour of such research did not differ significantly in their use of reasoned argument, in their dependence on authoritative pronouncement, in their reliance on established moral principle or in their recourse to dogmatic assertion. The advocates of embryo research were right to point out that most opposition to such research was linked to religious belief and justified, at least in part, on religious grounds. But religious discourse in the embryo debate was increasingly characterized by fragmentation, lack of certainty and toleration of conflicting interpretations, rather than by excessive dogmatism. It is true that some contributors denounced embryo research in the strongest terms as a threat to the Christian way of life and maintained this negative stance unwaveringly throughout the debate. However, other speakers with equally firm religious convictions supported embryo research from the outset; while many who initially opposed embryo research on religious grounds eventually changed their minds and came to regard such research as entirely compatible with their religious beliefs.

The parliamentary victory achieved by those in favour of embryo research was due less to the religious dogmatism of their opponents than to the collapse of unified religious opposition under pressure from the scientific lobby. As the debate proceeded, it became increasingly difficult for opponents of embryo research to insist that such research was contrary to Christian principle when other Christians saw it as in accord with the essential message of the scriptures, or as part of God's plan for the betterment of human society.[65] Opposition to embryo research was weakened by the absence of consistent religious leadership and by divisions within religious opinion which made religious condemnation of research on human embryos appear increasingly arbitrary. Religious opposition to embryo research was put under strain by the success of the scientific community in persuading lay people to accept both its account of the human embryo and its claims concerning the benefits of such research. Parliamentarians increasingly saw themselves as faced with a choice between sacrificing therapeutic benefits on a massive scale in defence of religious principles that were open to various conflicting interpretations, and adopting the scientists' view of the early embryo and, thereby, setting in motion a cumulative process of scientific and medical advance.

The scientific and medical communities were unified in their support for embryo research. Their members did not claim the right or the expertise to pronounce authoritatively on the moral questions arising from such research. But scientists, both individually and collectively, stated repeatedly that the early human embryo could be shown not to be a biological individual. These statements carried the clear implication that such embryos do not have the moral status of a person, and fall beyond the protective embrace of the principle of the sanctity of human life. The representatives of science also emphasized that the early embryo is an indispensable resource in the search for a wide range of medical benefits.

The resultant image of the early human embryo as a primitive organic entity lying outside the human community proper and available for utilitarian exploitation became the fundamental dogma of the pro-research movement. This belief can be described as a 'dogma' because it was universally endorsed by those in favour of embryo research; because it was regarded as unquestionably true on the basis of scientific authority; and because those who refused to accept this truth were often treated as irrational and/or as members of a separate moral community. Thus, in the course of the debate, widespread opposition to embryo research on the basis of a dogmatic interpretation of religious principle was gradually replaced by widespread approval of such research on the basis of a similarly dogmatic interpretation of the findings of science.

The 'dogma of the early embryo', although it was often presented as a neutral description of biological phenomena, arose directly out of the bitter struggle over the fate of embryo research, and contained evaluative as well as observational elements.[66] Similarly, scientists' claims about the future outcomes of embryo research, by their very nature, went well beyond the established facts. A few opponents tried to challenge the vision of a future in which research on human embryos would generate an endless supply of therapeutic benefits. It was suggested, for example, that genetic screening procedures were seldom successful when applied to large populations, and that scientists' promises concerning the potential benefits of embryo research would require the introduction of screening on a scale that could not be sustained. In other words, they argued that many of the most important benefits that were being cited to justify embryo research would turn out to have been illusory.[67]

Such warnings, however, were disregarded. Indeed, the difficulties of implementing effective IVF screening were never examined in detail. The great majority of parliamentarians simply chose to trust the scientific experts and to assume that, although there would inevitably be difficulties and setbacks, the scientific community would be able to keep its promises. Support for embryo research was based on the assumption that leading scientists and the scientific authorities could know what the future had in store. In the words of Lady Warnock: 'There can be no doubt about the goods that will flow from allowing the research to continue.'[68] Support for embryo research was based, to a considerable degree, on trusting acceptance of scientists' authoritative pronouncements and on faith in the ultimate benevolence of science.[69]

This chapter began with consideration of the claim that opposition to embryo research was due to the persistence of religious dogma, the resilience of religious faith and the power of religious authority. It has concluded with the proposal that reliance on dogma, authority and faith was as characteristic of the public discourse associated with science as it was of the discourse associated with religion. The material examined above suggests that dogma, authority and faith are intrinsic neither to religion nor to science, but are characteristic of either discourse insofar as it is dominant within an adversarial context.

In the initial stage of widespread denunciation of embryo research, it was religious discourse that was dominant and that exhibited these features. In contrast, during the later stage of scientific supremacy, religious opinion became more open and tolerant, while dogma, authority and faith became increasingly evident in the language of those who supported embryo research. The members of the pro-research lobby, unlike their opponents, had access to a well-established cultural stereotype, formed in the course of earlier scientific victories over religious opposition,[70] which gave them the advantage of being able to portray themselves as the exclusive representatives of detached, rational thought. In practice, however, the pro-research lobby triumphed, not because of its supporters' superior rationality or their detached assessment of the facts, but because it succeeded in imposing on the debate the cultural authority of science, and of generating thereby a sufficient degree of dogmatic conviction and unquestioning faith about the morality and benefits of embryo research among the decision-makers in Parliament.

8

The myth of Frankenstein

When people are faced with the task of making judgments about new areas of scientific inquiry, they are obliged to try to look into the future.[1] Given the inherent dynamism of science, people have to ask, not only whether the research in question is acceptable now, but also whether it will still be acceptable when it reaches maturity, and whether or not its immediate, practical benefits will be overshadowed by its wider, long-term consequences. This was clearly true of the debate over embryo research. The debate arose, in part, from the existence of differing opinions about the nature of the early human embryo and about the morality of conduct that requires the destructive use of such embryos. But the debate also involved a fundamental clash between different visions of what would happen in the future if human embryos were to continue to be employed for the purposes of scientific research.

Two figures of mythic dimensions were brought into play by participants in the debate as they attempted to convey, and to justify, their particular visions of the future. The first of these was the historical figure of Galileo. Galileo, as we have seen, entered the debate as a scientific martyr. Galileo's story was used to speak of the dangers of allowing people's non-scientific beliefs to impede the advance of scientific knowledge. Galileo was used to emphasize the human cost of outside interference of this kind. Galileo was one element in a pro-research rhetoric that was built around an optimistic vision of a future in which controlled research involving early human embryos would generate a cumulative series of major improvements in medical care, without contravening basic values or disrupting the fabric of social life.

The second mythic figure to appear in the debate was the fictional character of Dr Frankenstein. Frankenstein's role was, of course, that of the scientific villain. Frankenstein stood as a warning of the dangers inherent in scientists' ruthless and unending pursuit of knowledge. The tale of Frankenstein spoke, not of a world made better by science, but of the monstrous changes that would inevitably follow if scientists were allowed to step beyond the boundary of legitimate conduct and to use living human individuals as experimental subjects.

It may, at first, seem odd that the unreal world of science fiction should have become mixed up in this debate over serious issues of science policy. However, when people speculate about the development of new, science-based technologies, they cannot rely entirely on what they take to be the established facts. In thinking and arguing about the shape of things to come, they have no alternative but to create some kind of story which goes beyond these facts. Consequently, in the course of public appraisal of science and technology, the conventional boundary between fact and fiction may sometimes become blurred. In searching for the overall form of a real-life story which is at present incomplete, those involved must either invent a new, yet plausible, story-line or fit developments into a narrative structure that is already available. There is good reason, therefore, to expect that some of those who participate in public debate on such matters will turn to those fictional treatments of science that have become part of our common cultural repertoire. In addition, in the case of embryo research, there is an obvious parallel between Frankenstein's fictional creation of a living human being and Edwards and Steptoe's bestowal of life upon Louise Brown; and between the modern infertility clinic and the human production systems of Huxley's *Brave New World*.[2] These clear narrative similarities make it relatively easy to complete the unfinished test-tube baby plot with a story-line taken from science fiction.

The analytical literature on *Frankenstein*[3] and on other 'mad scientist' stories supports the supposition that these fictional products are relevant, in various ways, to happenings in the real world. Andrew Tudor, for example, in his cultural history of the horror film, argues that these texts map our landscapes of fear concerning science and provide evidence of 'changing popular images of what is threatening about science and scientists'.[4] He describes in detail how both the stories employed in such films and the moral lessons they convey have changed in response to alterations in the social location of scientists and to changes in the institutional uses of scientific knowledge.[5] Films about mad scientists, he maintains, beginning with the archetypical figure of Frankenstein, are expressions of a long-standing cultural ambivalence about science in which general recognition of the power of science is accompanied by a persistent fear of the terrible consequences that may follow when scientists' obsessive, amoral curiosity leads them to trespass in forbidden areas of inquiry.

A similar conclusion is reached in C. P. Toumey's examination of mad science fictions. Toumey argues that many, perhaps all, mad scientist stories are presented and interpreted, not just as enjoyable fantasies, but also as serious warnings about science and scientists. They operate, he suggests, as crude, yet memorable reminders of the ever-present possibility that scientists, by the very nature of their activities, may get things disastrously wrong and that ordinary people may suffer as a result.

Stories of mad scientists, whether textual or cinematic, constitute an extremely effective antirationalist critique of science. They thrill their audiences by brewing together suspense, horror, violence, and heroism and by uniting those features under the premise that most scientists are dangerous. Untrue, perhaps; preposterous, perhaps; low-brow, perhaps. But nevertheless effective.[6]

It follows from this kind of analysis that the narrative structures available in the mad scientist genre will be used regularly in the course of public debate concerning new, science-based technologies. Indeed, it will be precisely in those cases where some widely discussed scientific innovation has occurred which has practical consequences as yet unclear that the stories derived from anti-science fiction will be most relevant. For these fictions will work as effective warnings only if people use them for rhetorical purposes in cases of genuine uncertainty about the character of scientific research and the nature of its social impact.

We would not expect, of course, that the plots of specific books or films will normally be applied in detail to any particular area of scientific inquiry. The process of cultural transferral will usually operate more flexibly than this and the correspondence between fictional text and real-world extrapolation will often be more metaphorical than literal. Nevertheless, despite the potential variability of the process, there are strong grounds for expecting science fiction imagery to appear in debates such as that concerned with the development of embryo research. However, we must not take for granted that the resources of science fiction are available only to those who wish to attack or to restrain scientific development. As we shall see in the sections that follow, there is a fundamental weakness in science fiction imagery which enables the advocates of science to make Frankenstein and company speak in vigorous defence of the scientific enterprise.

Frankenstein in the press

The image of Frankenstein, or other fictional representations of scientific conduct, may appear in people's ordinary discourse in two different ways. In the first place, Frankenstein or his equivalents may be mentioned openly in relation to a serious issue such as the experimental manipulation of human IVF embryos. Secondly, participants may note the presence of fictional components in the discourse of other parties even though the latter may have made no explicit reference to the world of science fiction. Both these kinds of linkage between the realms of fact and fiction can be found in the debate over embryo research. Let us begin with an instance in which Frankenstein is clearly evident.

In November 1987, the Government presented its provisional framework for legislation concerning embryo research and the new reproductive technology.[7] This document made it clear that, if Parliament did grant permission for the continuation of research involving human IVF embryos, researchers would nevertheless be closely regulated by statute and subject to criminal sanctions. Two of the mass circulation newspapers responded with articles that contained explicit reference to Frankenstein and his monstrous creation. In the *Sun*, there was a still from the film *Frankenstein* accompanied by a brief account of the main recommendations contained in the White Paper.[8] *Today* published a similar item which began in the following way:

CLAMP ON FRANKENSTEIN SCIENTISTS
SCIENTISTS are to be banned by law from creating superbeings in the laboratory.
    The technique known as cloning, which can produce identical humans from a single cell, will also be made a criminal offence.
    The Government admits that the prospect of Frankenstein-style experiments is unlikely, but it wants to stop any genetic tinkering with embryos which would predetermine characteristics.
    A White Paper published yesterday proposes the clampdown on test-tube baby experiments.[9]

In both newspapers, the Frankenstein image dominated the text and was used to single out and to endorse the proposal to establish strict control over the activities of those scientists engaged in research on human embryos. By representing these scientists and their experiments in Frankensteinian terms, the newspapers seemed to imply that the former were potential malefactors; that if the legislative clamp were not applied, unfortunate consequences would follow – as in the fictional tale. There was a tension in both articles between the dramatic science fiction imagery and the official statements that Frankenstein-style experiments were 'unlikely' or 'extremely remote'. But these more modest assessments of the threat posed by embryo research were presented, unlike Frankenstein, without emphasis. Thus, the articles drew particular attention to the supposed resemblance between embryo researchers and Mary Shelley's scientific anti-hero. Frankenstein's prominence suggested strongly to readers that, despite official disclaimers, these scientists were dangerous and must be held on a tight rein.[10]

We cannot know how these articles were received by the newspapers' regular customers. We do know, however, that they were seen from within the scientific community as a characteristically ill-informed attack upon embryo research and upon science more generally. Thus, in *New Scientist*, the tactics adopted by the *Sun* were condemned in the editorial column as sensationalist and misleading.[11] Similarly *Nature*, in its news section, took the unusual step of reproducing the Frankenstein headline from *Today* by means of photo-montage and of adding the brief, contemptuous, comment: 'The popular press in Britain promotes a less than flattering view of scientists. *Today*'s response to last week's white paper.'[12] From the perspective of those sympathetic to embryo research, these articles in the popular press provided a clear illustration of the open, explicit use of the Frankenstein image to convey a critical message about the researchers investigating human embryos. The message was taken to be: 'Beware of science!'[13]

The appearance of negative, science fiction imagery in the debate over embryo research has provoked strong reactions from scientists. Robert Edwards, for example, has argued that such imagery has permeated public discussion of this topic and that much of the opposition to research on human embryos has been a direct result of the malign influence of science fiction.

If there are disagreements about the donation or freezing of human embryos, far greater passions are aroused about the need to carry out research on them. Everyone knows in principle that medical advances are built on scientific research, but the necessity or otherwise for experiments on human embryos sparks the most intense argument, as fears arise about tailor-made babies, or clones, or cyborgs, or some other nightmarish fancy.

The trouble really started way back in the 1930s, by courtesy of the brilliant Aldous Huxley. In his novel *Brave New World* . . . Admittedly some of Huxley's notions have come true. Fifty ova can now be collected from a human ovary. This is a modest figure compared with his thousands, yet his ideas still grip prophets of doom more than any other science fiction, as the numbers of human embryos growing in vitro rise year by year, and as his fellow writers whip up forebodings dire enough to alarm even the most phlegmatic science watcher. Whatever today's embryologists may do, Frankenstein or Faust or Jekyll will have foreshadowed, looming over every biological debate.[14]

Edwards offers here a general account of the underlying processes of the debate over embryo research in which his opponents are portrayed as responding, not to the modest, unthreatening realities of actual research, but to the exaggerated, misleading inventions of the fictional realm. We are invited to see their rejection of embryo research as arising from a confusion between illusion and reality. According to this interpretation, science fiction has had a significant but regrettable impact on the public debate in which Edwards has been involved. For it has tended to distort people's perception of where research on human embryos will lead and has generated fear and antagonism instead of fostering a proper appreciation of the benefits that further research will bring.[15]

Edwards's emphasis on the role played by science fiction in the debate operates as a defence of embryo research by removing its opponents' objections from the sphere of fact to the cognitively inferior domain of fiction. Because, in Edwards's view, these opponents are attacking the fantasies of the science fiction writers rather than the actualities of embryo research, their criticisms need not be taken seriously. These criticisms, like the fictional texts from which they are said to derive, come to be seen as a form of imaginary discourse. In contrast, Edwards's own assertions are presented as straightforwardly factual in character: 'In fact, of course, despite all the horror stories, most people connect embryo research with the early diagnosis or treatment of crippling diseases and therefore will concede, if pressed, that such research has been, and will continue to be, of great benefit to humanity.'[16] In this passage, Edwards seems to suggest that the horror stories of the science fiction writers have not, after all, *really* misled people; that, at some basic level, most of them recognize that embryo research is a good thing. Nevertheless elsewhere, as we have seen, he emphasizes that the stories of Huxley, Shelley and others have greatly affected public reactions to research involving human embryos and that they continue to 'loom over' embryologists' activities. In the first quotation above and in much of the subsequent discussion, he maintains unequivocally that the bulk of the opposition to embryo research has been built around images of *Brave New World* laboratories, Frankensteinian monsters and other science fiction fantasies.

If this line of argument is correct, we should expect to find that science fiction imagery appeared regularly in newspapers such as the *Sun* and *Today*, and in a good proportion of press items expressing criticism of embryo research. However, during the period for which I have systematic evidence of press coverage, that is, from December 1989 until the passage of the Human Fertilization and Embryology Act, this is not the case. In the first place, although more than thirty of the eighty-five items in my collection of press features[17] were critical of embryo research, only one made explicit use of the literature of science fiction. This feature consisted of four paragraphs taken from Huxley's *Brave New World* under the title 'Brave new embryos'.[18] The chosen passage, which had also been quoted by Edwards to illustrate the relevance of Huxley's novel to the current debate, deals with the mass production of human embryos. This item seems to be

an ironic comment on the long-term implications of the official endorsement of embryo research. But no attempt was made in the newspaper to use
this fictional fragment as the basis for open criticism of embryo research or
of the technology of assisted reproduction.

Furthermore, during the final phase of public debate, the mass-circula-
tion dailies such as the *Sun* and *Today* did not employ the kind of negative,
science fiction imagery that had appeared in response to the White Paper.
As we saw in chapter 5, they concentrated instead on the positive outcomes
of embryo research, and repeatedly built their stories around favourable
images of happy mothers holding healthy, contented, IVF babies. This
emphasis throughout the concluding stage of debate on the benefits of
embryo research shows that the earlier adoption of Frankensteinian
imagery was not part of a campaign of sustained opposition to such
research. The popular press was not imprisoned within the anti-science
rhetoric of science fiction, but seems to have been prepared to employ whatever resources were available to create dramatic headlines and newsworthy
stories.[19] Consequently, as the pro-research lobby became increasingly well
organized, the press coverage of embryo research came to be dominated,
not by science fiction imagery, but by the favourable images and story-lines
provided by the infertility clinics.

Science fiction imagery was almost entirely absent from the press during
the final phase of public debate over embryo research. Even those texts that
contained strong opposition to such research made no use of this kind of
imagery. Nevertheless, those sympathetic to embryo research continued to
voice the suspicion that Frankenstein and company were everywhere at
work and that their opponents were locked into an unreal world of monsters and mad scientists. For example, *New Scientist* opened its campaign
in support of embryo research at the start of the final sequence of parliamentary debate with a mocking denial that 'any embryo researcher has
tried to produce a monster with bolts in its neck, horns on its head or a
pointed tail'.[20] Later, as the decisive parliamentary vote approached, Dr
Bolton, an embryologist and 'chairman of Progress, an organization supporting research', was quoted in the *Mirror* as saying: 'We want to allay
public fears and prejudices that are perhaps compounded by those who
oppose us. We are not mad scientists. We want to alleviate suffering.'[21] On
both these occasions, of course, it was the advocates of embryo research
who actually made explicit use of science fiction imagery.

There is little evidence in the material examined so far to support the
claim advanced by Edwards and by other advocates of embryo research
that their critics' arguments were built around the 'mad scientist' fantasies
of the fictional realm. We must not forget, however, that the public

appraisal of embryo research occurred over a period of years and that critical use of science fiction imagery could have been more significant during earlier stages of debate. It is possible, for instance, that use of such imagery came to seem less appropriate to critics of embryo research once it had become clear that the new proposals introduced in the White Paper would formally prohibit those types of research that seemed most likely to lead directly towards genetic engineering. It is necessary, therefore, to ascertain how science fiction imagery was used during the initial phase of confrontation that preceded the White Paper. In order to do this, I shall turn to the parliamentary debates that followed the publication of the official report of the Warnock Committee.

Frankenstein in parliament

The opponents of embryo research dominated the early parliamentary debates until the tide began to turn in 1988. If science fiction imagery was crucial to the interpretative processes of organized opposition to embryo research, we would expect it to have been evident in the course of these debates. There were, however, only four instances in the five major debates between 1984 and 1988 where people opposed to embryo research openly used elements taken from science fiction. In two of them, reference was made to Huxley's *Brave New World* and in the other two, to some version of *Frankenstein*. The following speaker, for instance, begins the main part of her speech with these words: 'I once watched a science fiction film about a man who was made in a laboratory. He escaped and did all kinds of terrible things. It makes me think: is this the start of something which could lead to a Hitler theory of only the perfect human beings being brought into our society?'[22] She goes on to comment on the decline of Christianity, on the problems arising from abortion and childlessness, on the need to protect embryos from the moment of fertilization and on the usefulness of IVF in certain circumstances. In the middle section of her speech, she considers what she regards as the very real dangers of embryo research in a way that broadly parallels the earlier reference to the mythical laboratory of science fiction. 'The temptations for experimentation on the human embryo could go far,' she says. Scientists 'might try to reach their goal without regard to the embryo'. How, she asks, could we non-experts control them? Her overall conclusion is that embryo research should not continue and that 'the further we get away from nature, the more problems we shall have'.[23]

It appears that this speaker is drawing on some vague memory of a Frankenstein horror film in order to give form to her condemnation of this new type of research involving the laboratory production of human beings.

She uses a crude, minimal formulation of the Frankenstein story to convey the idea that the unanticipated consequences of this act of scientific trespass, difficult though they are to specify at this stage, may be most unwelcome. Her speech resembles the *Today* article in introducing fictional material explicitly into its appraisal of embryo research and in using the negative tone of the Frankenstein image to hint at the dangers that would follow if research in this area were allowed to continue.

Frankenstein is present in this first example from parliamentary debate, but his image is by no means dominant. The same is true of the passage below, taken from a later debate in the Commons in which Powell's Private Member's Bill is being discussed. The speaker asks the question: why is research on human embryos necessary? The scientists' answer, he claims, is that it is necessary because it will enable them eventually to control the processes of human reproduction and to eliminate genetic defects. This supposed reply generates a second rhetorical question:

Where are we going? If we take the rectification of genetic defects to its logical conclusion, one day we shall live in a society in which medical developments applied to *in vitro* fertilization will be so advanced that facial appearance, physical strength, skin colouring, IQ and intelligence will all have become the subject of laboratory experiment, so much so that one will be able to book an embryological configuration – tall, dark, handsome, short, intelligent, athletic, shrewd or perhaps even a Frankenstein monster if that is what one wants.[24]

Frankenstein is less central to this speech than to the articles in the popular press or to the speech quoted earlier. The reference to Frankenstein is not used here to establish the interpretative context, but appears to be added almost as an afterthought to the list of possible configurations. Yet Frankenstein's presence does contribute to our understanding of what is being said. It is the mention of Frankenstein that indicates most clearly in this part of the speech that the speaker is not simply offering a neutral description of what he thinks is likely to happen, but is also expressing his disapproval and repugnance. In other words, Frankenstein's introduction works to imply a moral resemblance between the fictional scientist's monstrous achievement and the excesses to be expected of real scientists in the foreseeable future.

Although Frankenstein is employed by this speaker to signal that he is appalled by the prospect of continued research on human embryos, the reference to science fiction is not essential to the speech. The speaker's account of the science-based technology of the future derives textually, not from the Frankenstein myth, but from his imaginative reconstruction of the discourse of actual scientists at work today. Frankenstein plays only a peripheral role in these speculations. As with the previous speaker, reference to the fictional character seems to be little more than a convenient device with which to convey negative feelings and a sense of apprehension about the direction in which certain sectors of modern science appear to be heading. The same is true of participants' occasional use of *Brave New World* for critical purposes.

The public will want some specific questions answered exactly. For example, how can we get sufficient numbers of sufficiently qualified scientific inspectors to differentiate between a 14-day and a 15-day old embryo . . . ? The public will want proper answers to those . . . questions. There are widespread, and I believe well-informed, fears lest trans-species fertilization lead beyond embryonic growth to a mixed breed, converting the uniqueness of man into a bastardized freak. The public, I believe, will revolt against debasement of human generation to stud farming methods. I believe that the public is already showing signs of an instinctive resistance to the Brave New World's intrusion into this most private and sacred area of human experience.[25]

These examples show that parliamentary critics of embryo research did sometimes refer to science fiction in their attempts to speculate about the future and to demonstrate the need, either to ban such research or to exercise greater control over scientists' activities. But we could hardly conclude, from occasional, passing references of this kind, that science fiction had exerted a major influence on the opposition party. Indeed, negative science fiction imagery was actually used more frequently in these debates by the supporters of embryo research than by its critics.[26] We find, however, as in the material discussed in the previous section, that advocates of embryo research claimed to be able to detect Frankenstein's influence upon their opponents whether or not these opponents happened to mention him.

We are provided with opportunities for alleviating the miseries and problems that infertility inflicts on individuals and society and, at the same time, letting loose upon society the forces that could do more harm than good. I cannot help feeling that Mary Shelley's spectre of Dr Frankenstein's monster impinges heavily on our subconscious when we address ourselves to the problem of embryology, causing a fear of and revulsion against the possible products of the ruthless pursuit of knowledge for its own sake or the application of medical techniques to create monsters or superhumans.[27]

The speaker continues by acknowledging that the idea of Frankenstein's monster may have some value if it encourages people to 'be on their guard' and to ensure that the new science-based techniques are not improperly used. Nevertheless, he insists, we must not let our powerful feelings of fear and revulsion prevent us from recognizing and accepting the benefits that controlled embryo research will bring. We must not, he implies, make the mistake of taking Mary Shelley's story too literally. We must instead do our best to control the Frankenstein-inspired promptings of our subconscious minds and to avoid adopting uncritically the negative preconceptions evident in so many contributions to the public debate. In this speaker's view, although we are all influenced by the Frankenstein myth, some people have been able to restrain that influence and to deal with the issues under review in a more detached and logical manner. Such an approach, he contends, leads to cautious support for the use of IVF and for the continuation of embryo research.

A similar assessment of Frankenstein's significance in the public debate over embryo research is proposed by another pro-research speaker in the same parliamentary session. Embryo research, he says, 'is a subject fraught with fantasies of futuristic horror. Lurid associations with "Brave New World" embryology, Nazi medicine or Frankenstein experimentation, make debate between irreconcilable moral positions very difficult.'[28] Belief in these horror stories is said to make debate difficult because it is associated with a stance of such moral certitude that rational discussion becomes impossible. As he puts it in a later session, one of the major obstacles preventing dispassionate debate 'is the dread that scientists are somehow running amok and that unless they are reined in by immediate legislation, science fiction nightmares such as human–hamster hybrids, carbon copy cloning by nuclear transplantation or wanton torture of living fetuses in the laboratory might see the light of day'.[29]

Once again, Frankenstein and company are portrayed as having prevented the critics of embryo research from properly grasping its realities. In contrast, for those who, like the speaker, are able to step outside the realm of fantasy and to avoid the moral absolutism justified by its imaginary horrors, 'the benefits of controlled research, closely monitored and regulated by a licensing body of the sort recommended by the Warnock committee, seem to be compelling'.[30] It will be evident that this use of science fiction imagery closely resembles pro-researchers' references to religious dogmatism. In both cases, speakers seek to undermine the testimony of those opposed to embryo research by removing their arguments from the factual realm to an unreliable, non-factual domain of supposition, fantasy and mere belief.[31]

In the course of the embryo debate, in Parliament and in the media, negative science fiction imagery was used explicitly by supporters of embryo research as well as by its critics. For the latter, science fiction was available as a convenient cultural resource with which to convey disapproval and apprehension. For the former, it was a resource with which to weaken the credibility of their opponents' speculations about the future and to explain away their refusal to accept the reassurances offered by the representatives of scientific research. When Frankenstein appeared within the context of anti-research discourse, he reminded recipients forcefully of the potential dangers of scientific development. When Frankenstein appeared within the context of pro-research discourse, he was made to speak, along with Galileo, not of the dangers of science, but of the credulity, ignorance and dogmatism of those who were unwilling to support the advance of scientific knowledge.[32]

Competing visions of the future

The material presented above has one puzzling feature; namely, how was it possible for scientists and other supporters of embryo research to insist that science fiction was a major influence on their opponents, when those opponents made little explicit use of science fiction imagery? It is clear that explicit reference to science fiction was not essential for its influence to be detected. At least some of those in favour of embryo research were able to infer the influence of Frankenstein and of science fiction more generally from other, less obvious, features of their opponents' arguments in relation to embryo research. Let me examine one parliamentary speech in which these features can be observed. In order to illustrate the full range of characteristics involved, I will quote at length from this speech:

I want to consider where this whole matter will lead us . . . Ectogenesis involves maintaining the embryo *in vitro* for progressively longer periods. Why have a limit of 14 days? Why should it not be extended to 20, 30 or 40 days? The ultimate goal may be to produce a child entirely *in vitro* or to produce genetically identical individuals by cloning. In other words, the goal may be to mimic the natural process leading to selective breeding or the creation of human beings with predetermined characteristics . . . One can see that coming, not in a lifetime but in two lifetimes. All those matters are hypothetical, but they may come about. As we are aware, we slide from one piece of primary legislation and so on . . . I now want to consider trans-species investigations. We are all aware that in agriculture they have combined a sheep and a goat and a rather remarkable beast was formed. It would not take a great leap of imagination to imagine what might happen. Each cell has its DNA. It is possible through genetic engineering and manipulation of cells to remove or to splice in a link and that might have catastrophic consequences . . . The White Paper . . . says that we must have a system of mandatory licensing. The system would, of course, create a criminal offence. But . . . most of the activities in breach of the law could be compiled clandestinely. Therefore, while one might get the respect of those who have respect for the law, those who thirst for knowledge, regardless of restraint, will work unceasingly for what they term their aspirations . . . The dignity of man must remain inviolate. His status is degraded as soon as the legislature permits us to interfere, to man's detriment, with any part of his being, whether in time of growth or synthesis . . . There have been great achievements throughout British medicine and I pay tribute to the work that has been done. Having said all that, surely we in the House can see, down the labyrinth of years, the dangers to which we are exposed, and the dangers to which we are exposing the nation.[33]

This speaker, like so many opposed to embryo research, formulates his response on the basis of what he takes to be its long-term consequences. Where will it lead us, he asks, not in one lifetime, but across the span of generations to come? He recognizes that, in attempting to look so far ahead, he must rely on his imagination. But he treats disciplined extrapolation from what is known about present-day science as a necessary and legitimate part of the process of appraisal.

In his imaginative vision of a future in which research on human embryos has been allowed to continue, the speaker attributes great power to science. He assumes, in particular, that scientists will sooner or later succeed in their attempts to mimic and control the natural mechanisms of human reproduction. However, this acknowledgement of scientists' potency is combined with a profound distrust. A significant proportion of scientists, he suggests, will pursue their technical objectives without respect for the law or for the fundamental values on which human dignity depends. He seems to imply that it is the very amorality of scientific culture that makes it so technically successful, yet at the same time so resistant to external regulation.[34] He concludes, therefore, that technical accomplishments such as sexual selection, cloning, genetic manipulation, trans-species fertilization, and so on, which are at the moment either hypothetical or in their infancy, furnish faint but prophetic clues to the achievements of the future and to the disruptive social changes that will in due course follow if scientists are permitted to continue their inquiries in the realm of human creation.

This type of abstract narrative appeared repeatedly throughout the parliamentary campaign against embryo research.[35] Its characteristic elements are the extended temporal perspective, the open dependence on imaginative work, the suspicious recognition of the power of science, the stress placed on scientists' obsessive pursuit of technical goals, the emphasis on the difficulty of controlling science from outside, the significance attributed to certain unusual technical developments in contemporary science, and the expression of repugnance at scientists' incursion into a sacred region of human existence.

Although the original Frankenstein story and its fictional derivatives employ much more concrete and particularized story-lines than does the speaker above, there are numerous parallels between the two kinds of narrative structure. In the first instance, both types of narrative take place outside the time-span of ordinary experience; that is, they occur either in a fictional recreation of the past or in an as yet unrealized future. Secondly, the typical anti-science fiction and critical speculation concerning the development of embryo research are both built around a 'generalized fear that the engine of change is out of control'.[36] Scientists' motives tend to be depicted in both these kinds of text as untrustworthy and as leading them to trespass, with disastrous results, in forbidden areas.[37] Thus, thirdly, scientists are seen as ignoring the limitations implied by commonly accepted values and, consequently, as threatening irreparable damage to the social fabric.[38] The science fiction horror film and the denunciatory prophecy about embryo research can be seen to be similar in kind because they are both creative projections of negative assumptions about science and about scientists. It is the expression of these underlying assumptions *in an undeniably imaginative form* by the critics of embryo research that enabled those defending science to treat this type of supposedly real-world discourse as deriving from, and as implicitly belonging to, the genre of anti-science fiction.

It follows from this argument that explicit reference to the fictional realm was not required for opposition discourse to be seen as a form of anti-science fiction by supporters of embryo research. The negative representation of scientists' motives, the condemnation of scientific amorality and the temporal extension of the narrative line could in themselves be taken to reveal such discourse as unreal in character, irrespective of its detailed content. I suggest that it was the repeated appearance of these features in opposition rhetoric that led supporters of embryo research to conclude that Frankenstein and company were constantly at work behind the scenes.

Adoption of an extended temporal perspective was essential to opponents of embryo research because it created interpretative space in which they could exercise their critical imagination. It was only by looking well into the future that they were able to postulate dramatic technical changes and to envisage radically new forms of science-based activity which were clearly incompatible with present-day morality. Advocates of research regularly attacked their opponents' use of this temporal strategy and repeatedly urged that the discussion be kept 'undistorted by wild speculations' about the far distant future. In so doing, they reaffirmed the apparently more cautious approach employed in the Warnock Report of keeping the temporal perspective short, and reliance on imagination to a minimum.[39]

Despite their rejection of their opponents' speculative efforts as 'exaggerated and emotive propaganda'[40] and despite their commitment, in principle, to a policy of short-term realism, the supporters of embryo research, in practice, also made much use of imaginative claims about the future.[41] Let me offer just one illustration taken from a speaker whom we have seen above several times condemning other people's futuristic fantasies:

Research that holds the prospect of reducing this blight on so many lives must be welcomed. Moreover, such work can reduce the incidence of miscarriage . . . But the potential for research goes much wider. Information could emerge on how a range of birth defects arises or on how cancer cells become malignant. It may also help to remedy genetic disease, which affects one in 50 children . . . For the future – it may be a distant future, but it is foreseeable – it could be possible to use cells, which divide to form specific organs in the embryo, to correct blood disorders or repair damaged tissue in the pancreas or even the heart, the brain or the liver of an adult.[42]

Those in favour of embryo research, such as this speaker, regularly slipped into the prophetic mode; although, of course, their speculations concentrated on the expected benefits of such research rather than the problems to which it might give rise.[43] Such claims were often challenged. They were, however, never depicted as blatant fantasies deriving from the fictional realm. This was, presumably, because there was no well-known fictional genre to which such optimistic extrapolations could be linked.[44] Although both sides in the debate creatively projected their divergent conceptions of science into the future as a way of justifying their present course of action, the advocates of embryo research had the advantage of being able to maintain that their positive vision was supported by the authority of science. In contrast, those engaged in opposition to embryo research laboured under the disadvantage that their bleak narratives bore a distinct resemblance to certain familiar stories from science fiction. We cannot know for certain how these differing alignments in relation to the domains of science and science fiction affected the eventual outcome of the debate. Nevertheless, it seems likely, from what we have seen above, that the existence of a fictional genre expressing widespread fears about science and technology tended, somewhat paradoxically, to weaken the campaign against embryo research and to strengthen the arguments of those who spoke in its defence.

9

Embryo research and the slippery slope

I will begin this chapter with a summary of the reasons for the success in the parliamentary debate of those who supported embryo research.[1] The major outcome of this debate was the establishment of the Human Fertilization and Embryology Authority (HFEA) with responsibility for ensuring that research and clinical practice involving human IVF embryos in Britain is carried out in accordance with the regulations laid down in the 1990 Act, and for guiding the further development of embryo research. In the next two sections, I shall examine some of the cultural tensions facing the HFEA as it attempts to fulfil these obligations. I shall then compare the system of regulation that has been adopted in Britain with the system under discussion in the USA, before concluding with some brief observations on the pattern of social change that is likely to occur in the years ahead.

The triumph of hope over fear

The pro-research lobby emerged victorious from the series of parliamentary confrontations that took place during the 1980s. It had succeeded, not only in attracting support from many politicians who had been undecided initially about the use of human embryos for experimental purposes, but also in gaining the votes of a substantial number of those who had at first been firmly opposed to research of this kind. This success was due to a combination of many different factors. The long delay in the introduction of the Government Bill was important because it gave time, not only for the formation of an organized pro-research lobby, but also for the lobby's campaign of persuasion to take effect. The inclusion of clauses clearly forbidding genetic engineering in the Government's White Paper helped to reduce the level of parliamentary anxiety about the long-term consequences of embryo research and made parliamentarians more receptive to arguments in favour of its continuation. The creation of the Voluntary Licensing Authority was a significant factor because scientists' co-operation with the VLA was widely taken as showing that embryo research could be properly monitored and regulated by the kind of statutory agency recommended in the Warnock Report.

The success of the pro-research lobby was also due to the control exercised by the infertility clinics over the stories and imagery presented in the media; to the development of a potent rhetoric in which moving personal narrative was combined with expert scientific testimony; to the skilful use of parliamentary tactics and external pressure groups; to the policy of fostering direct contact between parliamentarians and practising scientists; to the strong endorsement of embryo research by female representatives during the final phase of debate; to the forceful use of cultural stereotypes by supporters of embryo research to weaken the credibility of their opponents; and to the striking contrast between religious fragmentation and scientific unity.

It will be clear from previous chapters that, to some extent, the anti-research lobby contributed to its own defeat by a number of tactical failures.[2] For example, its members made little attempt to extend or to revise their basic position as the debate proceeded, but relied heavily on constant repetition of the abstract moral arguments taken over from the anti-abortion movement. In addition, although they complained frequently about their adversaries' manipulation of the media, they do not seem to have tried to reduce their opponents' dominance in the media by drawing attention there to the many instances in which women suffered from their exposure to the techniques of assisted reproduction. Nor did they use the personal testimony of such women in Parliament to try to reveal the utopian assumptions underlying the pro-research rhetoric of hope.

Each of these factors played a part in the triumph of the pro-research lobby. They did so by contributing to three critical changes in parliamentarians' conception of embryo research. The most fundamental of these was the transformation of participants' understanding of the experimental subject of embryo research. At the beginning of the debate, most parliamentary speakers insisted that such research was immoral because it involved experimental manipulation of defenceless human individuals. By the end of the debate, most speakers maintained that experimental activity in this field was legitimate because it was, and would continue to be, confined to a minute collection of cells called the 'pre-embryo' which preceded the emergence of the human individual. The idea of the 'pre-embryo' helped to remove the moral barrier to the continuation of embryo research by convincing people and/or by helping them to express their conviction that this was not research involving real human beings, but experimental use of unformed biological material. This view came to be widely endorsed, clearly articulated and supported with a range of arguments furnished by the scientists. This flood of science-based argument tended to undermine and to negate the image of the embryo as an unborn human individual and, thereby, for many participants, to make irrelevant the moral rhetoric of personhood and rights. The great polemical advantage of the concept of the 'pre-embryo' for the pro-research lobby was that it placed the experimental subject of embryo research beyond the reach of its opponents' moral discourse.

The second crucial element in the success of the pro-research campaign was its increasing emphasis on the possibility of controlling genetic disease without altering the genetic make-up of human individuals. The pro-research lobby convinced the majority of parliamentarians that many forms of genetic disorder could be more or less eradicated by means of genetic screening of IVF embryos. As a result, as the parliamentary debate entered its concluding stage, the defenceless unborn children of the early debates largely disappeared from view and were replaced by the miraculously healthy children to be produced in due course with the techniques forthcoming from embryo research. The replacement of the embryo by the pre-embryo made further research seem permissible. The acceptance of scientists' claims concerning the wide range of potential benefits to be obtained by means of genetic screening made the continuation of embryo research appear obligatory to the majority of parliamentarians.

The third crucial element in the success of the pro-research lobby was its replacement of its opponents' rhetoric of fear concerning the long-term impact of embryo research with an alternative rhetoric of hope.[3] The critics of embryo research were fearful because, in their view, such research involved a fundamental moral transgression which would encourage further, yet more outrageous, forms of immoral conduct. They argued that approval of embryo research by Parliament would open the way for a steady expansion in the scope of scientific inquiry and in the impact of reproductive science on established patterns of social life. When they attempted to assess the results of such research, they saw much to cause them grave concern. Given their assumption that embryo research was itself intrinsically evil, it seemed obvious to them that its continued growth and technological exploitation would combine with wider historical processes to weaken the hold of civilized values.

The success of the pro-research lobby in convincing parliamentarians that embryo research was both permissible and medically valuable enabled its members to promote a much more optimistic vision of the future in which fear and anxiety gave way to confident anticipation of better things to come. In this alternative rhetoric, it was emphasized that the scientists engaged in embryo research enthusiastically supported the values of society at large and that their overriding aim was to produce results that would reduce suffering and increase people's access to normal family life. In the words of *New Scientist*, embryo research was 'the manipulation of nature for the purposes of Good'.[4] The rhetoric of justification adopted by the supporters of embryo research depicted a future in which a stream of beneficial consequences would flow from the organized production of new techniques for controlling the biological aspects of human reproduction. It was a future in which countless people would have a realistic hope of achieving a better life with the help of the practitioners of embryo research.

Both the rhetoric of hope and the rhetoric of fear were employed as resources in a fierce struggle for political supremacy. It was inevitable, therefore, that they would both be used to offer selective accounts of the social consequences of embryo research. The rhetoric of fear was intended to show that any benefits from embryo research would necessarily be overshadowed by the unanticipated and socially disruptive changes that would follow from increasing science-based control over the most intimate and personal areas of human experience. The rhetoric of the pro-research lobby, on the other hand, tended to focus narrowly on the provision of technical solutions to medical problems and to ignore the wider social and economic context. The rhetoric of hope was built around the implicit assumption that the scientific community could guarantee major advances in medical therapy and that these technical accomplishments could be transformed into improvements in social welfare without producing unanticipated or unwelcome social by-products. The pro-research lobby argued that the evolution of embryo research and the application of its technological products could be controlled by the creation of an external statutory agency. The opponents of embryo research insisted that any mechanism of external control would eventually be eroded by the internal dynamic of scientific inquiry and that, sooner or later, society's defences would be overrun. As we have seen, the majority of parliamentarians chose to reject the warnings of the anti-research lobby and to accept the reassuring image of embryo research as a powerful, yet obedient, servant of society.

The parliamentary debate ended with the formal approval of embryo research and with the establishment of the HFEA. The HFEA was given the task of ensuring that embryo research would continue to develop in ways that were medically beneficial, whilst also making sure that researchers and clinicians continued to act in a socially responsible manner. In its first annual report, the HFEA noted that research in relation to assisted conception 'is currently moving forward at a great pace'.[5] Readers were assured, however, that the Authority would try to anticipate and to address any new social or ethical issues arising from embryo research and assisted reproduction before they became urgent, and that it would attempt to resolve such issues with the help of informed and enlightened public debate. The HFEA, it was said, would 'work towards a steady and general point of view taking account of the Human Fertilization and Embryology Act and based on moral reasoning'.[6] In other words, the embryo debate of the 1980s was to continue into the new decade, and indeed into the new century, but from now on it would operate under the supervision of the HFEA and within the terms of reference built into the legislation approved by the parliamentary majority in 1990.

The divided embryo

Although the concept of the pre-embryo was central to the parliamentary victory of the pro-research lobby, the term 'pre-embryo' was not used in the Human Fertilization and Embryology Act. Nevertheless, the concept is implicit in the clauses that forbid scientists to keep or make use of a human IVF embryo beyond the first fourteen days or 'after the appearance of the primitive streak'.[7] These clauses are based on the assumption that the human embryo undergoes a fundamental change of status around day fourteen. They imply that, at this point in its development, the embryo becomes a human individual who must not be used for experimental purposes and who deserves our protection in accordance with the principle of the sanctity of each human life.[8]

The fourteen-day rule is meant to be an unequivocal expression of the judgment of the parliamentary majority concerning the proper limit to the use of human embryos for purposes of scientific inquiry. The rule is intended to ensure that pre-fourteen-day embryos are clearly distinguished from post-fourteen-day embryos and that both types of embryo are treated in a manner appropriate to their moral status. Its adoption, however, has created anomalous situations of two kinds. In the first place, it can be argued, there are circumstances in which human individuals may be treated as if they were 'pre-embryos'. Secondly, it can be argued that there are circumstances in which what are supposed to be 'pre-embryos' are regularly treated as if they were human individuals. Thus the embodiment of this new moral boundary in the 1990 Act has created a region of cultural ambiguity which is open to exploitation by those who are still opposed to embryo research.

The first potential anomaly arises because the Act states that scientists shall not keep or use an embryo *after the appearance of the primitive streak*. It seems to follow from this formulation that scientists are entitled to wait until experimental embryos have become human individuals before they are obliged to destroy them. Those who are sympathetic to embryo research might be inclined to dismiss this issue as a relatively trivial matter. They might reasonably observe that the appearance of the primitive streak is no more than the first minute step in the formation of a biologically organized individual organism. They might also point out that, at present, laboratory embryos do not survive the full fourteen days and, therefore, that the destruction of human organisms displaying a primitive streak does not yet occur in practice.

Those who are opposed to such research, however, regard this issue as more serious. They are inclined to insist that the Human Fertilization and Embryology Act is internally flawed because it allows flagrant violation of the new moral boundary which was supposed to provide a strict limit to scientists' use of human embryos. In the following quotation from a recent edition of *LIFE News*, we can see a member of the anti-abortion movement employing this form of argument in the course of a vigorous denunciation of the HFEA:

The 14-day time-limit for human embryos is in effect an order to execute. The law dictates that the passing of the fourteenth day confers 'humanity' on the embryo and requires that it be destroyed. The appearance of the primitive streak, so beloved of Anne McLaren and Mary Warnock, is both the moment when, allegedly, humanity appears and when the new human being must be destroyed – a strange fusion of ideas.[9]

This passage is more than a restatement of the basic anti-abortion claim that all human embryos should be treated as living persons. The author goes beyond this in asserting that the Human Fertilization and Embryology Act permits grossly improper treatment of beings who are defined as human individuals within the Act's own terms of reference. For this author and his like-minded readers, there is clear evidence here of moral inconsistency and, perhaps, of bad faith on the part of those responsible for controlling the conduct of embryo research.

The first cultural tension, then, arising from the formal establishment of the fourteen-day boundary is that it can reasonably be argued that entities which should be classed officially as human individuals could, under certain circumstances, be treated as if they were 'pre-embryos'. The second cultural tension is that entities that should be regarded officially as 'pre-embryos' may sometimes be treated as human individuals or, indeed, as unborn children. This reverse form of violation of the embryo/pre-embryo boundary is likely to occur quite frequently. The basic reason for this is that the clinical practice associated with embryo research brings its clients into close contact with living human organisms newly created outside the womb. Contact of this kind may encourage those clients to regard the cluster of cells in which they are personally interested as a human individual from the earliest stage of its biological development.

It has been shown that visual imaging techniques, such as ultrasound, can have this effect during later stages of non-IVF pregnancies by making the developing fetus look like an unborn child. This technically mediated access to the new human organism blurs the boundary between fetus and baby. It reinforces the idea that the emergent being exists as a separate, autonomous individual.[10] It seems likely that IVF techniques often work in a similar fashion to promote the view that the early embryo is already an identifiable human being. For example, when patients and doctors in infertility clinics use preimplantation genetic diagnosis to select between normal and abnormal embryos, they seem to be treating each separate embryonic organism as a potential person with recognizable attributes. Their choice undoubtedly involves a technical comparison between cellular clusters bearing different genetic configurations. Yet the choice also involves some conception of what kind of person each entity will be likely to become. It is, in this sense, a choice between human organisms which are seen as developing human individuals and also, perhaps, as prospective members of a specific human family.

However doctors, scientists and legislators define early human embryos for technical or for legal purposes, it is difficult to believe that potential parents do not often speak, and think, of them as unborn children. This view is clearly conveyed by the words of an enthusiastic IVF father who appeared in a recent television programme: 'It's pretty amazing, the fact that you get to see your child when the cell first splits. You actually get to see your child an hour after conception. I was elated. I thought that was the most – to see that child in the dish was the most amazing thing I've ever seen.'[11] In the following quotation, a woman born without a womb describes her distress as the person acting as her surrogate walked from the clinic pregnant with her two implanted IVF embryos: 'It was an awful moment. She was walking off with my babies and I was going to be miles away from them. It didn't matter where they were, they were still mine. My feelings towards them were no different from any other mother.'[12]

In both these cases, the individuals concerned developed a strong parental relationship with their pre-fourteen-day embryos. Thus it appears that, although the legal outcome of the parliamentary process embodies a rigid distinction between the human embryonic material deemed to exist during the first fourteen days after fertilization and the human individuals who appear subsequently, the medical practice deriving from embryo research actively fosters, at least for some participants on some occasions, an image of the early embryo as an individual person from the time of conception. It seems that the boundary implicit in the fourteen-day rule may be regularly ignored in the clinical context as would-be parents respond to the living products of IVF technology.

There is no evidence in the popular literature produced by the anti-abortion movement to suggest that its members are aware of the potential anomaly created by the appearance of 'unborn children' at the heart of assisted reproduction.[13] Nevertheless, it is clear that some members of the anti-abortion movement have assumed responsibility for monitoring the activities of the HFEA and of policing the moral boundary that derives from the concept of the pre-embryo.[14] One part of their strategy, as we saw in the passage from *LIFE News* quoted above, is to try to draw attention to those points of cultural tension that arise out of the implementation of this boundary. The characterization of early embryos as unborn children within the clinical context is one such point of tension. It is not, of course, formally incompatible with the requirements of the Human Fertilization and Embryology Act. But it would be possible to cite this phenomenon as an indication that many people within the infertility clinics adopt a view of the early human embryo that is difficult to reconcile with its use as an experimental subject. However, any observations or complaints made by the anti-abortion movement about actual or potential moral inconsistency in relation to the embryo/pre-embryo boundary are unlikely to have much impact, except among its own members. There are several reasons why this is so.

In the first place, those who are engaged in embryo research, or who are formally involved in its administration, will always be able to offer alternative interpretations of any apparent 'violations' of the boundary. For instance, talk about 'unborn children' in the infertility clinics could be explained away as being due to the understandable, but misguided, reactions of technically untrained people who were desperate for a child.[15] From the official perspective, references to children in Petri dishes would simply be regarded as lay persons' mistakes. Secondly, we saw in the examination of parliamentary debate that the anti-abortion movement came to be regarded by those responsible for implementing the 1990 Act as part of a separate moral community whose views on embryo research and related matters could be disregarded.[16] As a result, the movement has no representation on the HFEA and comments by its members on issues relating to the Act are routinely dismissed as irrelevant by that body.[17] In other words, the establishment of the HFEA and the transfer of debate outside the formal parliamentary setting have changed the balance of power to the disadvantage of the anti-abortion lobby. Thirdly, many of the questions concerning the treatment of early human embryos which are seen as morally significant by anti-abortionists are unlikely to attract interest from the media or from citizens unconcerned about the rights or moral status of the unborn. Yet, without such support from other 'legitimate' sectors of society, the politically marginalized anti-abortion movement will be unable to mount an effective challenge to the continuation of embryo research, to the actions of the official administrative agency, or to the existence of the embryo/pre-embryo boundary.

Support of this kind will be likely to occur only insofar as there are other cultural tensions that generate anxiety over embryo research and its products elsewhere in society. In the next section, I shall examine two major ethical issues which have been identified by the HFEA itself as in need of attention and which have given rise to considerable public concern, and to widespread debate.

The process of ethical control

During the first three years of its existence, the HFEA noted in its annual reports that there were various unanswered questions relating to embryo research and to the provision of infertility services which needed to be examined in terms of ethical, as well as practical, considerations. The Authority was uncertain, for example, whether payment of any kind should be made to the people who donate sperm or eggs; whether such donors should be allowed to remain anonymous; whether women should be allowed to choose the ethnic background of their egg or sperm donor; whether it is appropriate for post-menopausal women to be given infertility treatment; whether human embryos should be selected for implantation on the basis of their sex; and whether it is permissible to use eggs taken from aborted fetuses, or from other cadavers, for purposes of research and/or for purposes of assisted reproduction. These and other related issues were put forward for public scrutiny by the Authority in order to ensure that its members were aware of public opinion on these matters and to help ordinary people to understand the activities and formal decisions of the HFEA. In this section, I will consider how the Authority dealt with the issues of sex selection and the use of fetal and cadaveric eggs. These two examples will enable us to see how the process of ethical control set up in the 1990 Act operates in practice.

Implantation of IVF embryos that had been screened for sex was first accomplished in the UK in 1989 as a result of research undertaken at the Hammersmith Hospital by Robert Winston and his colleagues. Female embryos were selected in this instance in order to make sure that a life-threatening condition linked to the male chromosome could not be transmitted. This kind of use of IVF techniques for medical purposes was approved in the 1990 Act. The HFEA made clear in 1993 that 'selecting against all male embryos is a compromise measure'[18] which would become redundant when it became possible to identify, and to discard, those individual embryos that actually carry the faulty gene. In the meantime, however, another technique, designed to achieve sex selection by the separation of male from female sperm, had also become available. As a result, discussion had begun in the media and elsewhere about whether it was legitimate to allow people to choose the sex of their children, either by sperm sorting or by IVF methods. In January 1993, the HFEA issued a consultation document which was intended to clarify the current situation, to stimulate public discussion and to generate responses that would help the Authority to decide how best to regulate those techniques of sex selection that came under its control.

The consultation document emphasized that the HFEA had no doubts about the morality of sex selection for medical purposes. What needed to be decided, in the view of the Authority, was whether people should be allowed to try to choose the sex of a child 'for social reasons'.[19] No attempt was made to distinguish rigorously between 'medical' and 'social' reasons in the document. But examples of the latter were provided: 'A couple may want to have a girl or a boy for a variety of social reasons. For example, they may already have a child, or children, of one sex and would like one of the other or they may attach higher status to one sex rather than the other.'[20]

The Authority's document went on to furnish a series of moral arguments which might be used either to support or to condemn sex selection for social reasons. It was suggested, for instance, that some citizens might claim that the sexual composition of one's family was a private matter which should not be subject to outside regulation; or that children whose sex had been chosen would be loved with greater intensity than would children whose sex had been determined by chance and that, consequently, the overall quality of family life would be raised to a higher level by the use of techniques of sex selection. Alternatively, it was suggested that other people might argue, for example, that the use of these techniques would upset the natural balance of the sexes; or that approval of sex selection would start to propel society down a 'slippery slope' towards a situation in which only 'perfect babies' were acceptable. No attempt was made to assess the moral validity of the two opposing sets of arguments presented in the consultation document. Readers were invited to come to their own conclusions about sex selection and to let the HFEA know their views so that they could be taken into account.

The Authority distributed 2,000 copies of its consultation document and for the next four months the topic was widely discussed in the media and in other settings.[21] The public response was very similar to that which had initially greeted the Warnock Report in 1984; that is, sex selection for social reasons was overwhelmingly rejected. Some of the arguments used to condemn embryo research were reapplied to the new topic. However, opposition to the new techniques was not confined to those who had previously objected to the use of human embryos for purposes of research, but also came from some of those who had enthusiastically supported such research. The Archbishop of York, for example, wrote to *The Times* to try to persuade its readers that it would be wrong to use the results of embryo research to allow people freely to choose the sex of their offspring:

Babies are not products but persons, and because this distinction is so fundamental to our understanding of what human beings are, anything which might tend to blur it should be resisted . . . Embryo selection through IVF might be justified in the case of sex-linked hereditary diseases but should not, in my view, be acceptable for purely personal or social reasons.[22]

The Archbishop went on to maintain that the essential problem with uncontrolled sex selection lay in its long-term social consequences and, in particular, in its tendency to corrupt people's attitudes towards children. In other words, his Lordship had come to the conclusion that this use of IVF techniques had to be stopped because it would be a clear step down the slippery slope of moral decline that had so concerned his opponents during the parliamentary debates of the previous decade.

Although the consultation document succeeded in stimulating public discussion over sex selection, the formal response was disappointing and the HFEA received only a few hundred written replies.[23] Nevertheless, once the period of public appraisal had ended, a firm statement was quickly issued to the effect that 'the Authority is persuaded by the arguments against sex selection for social reasons and this view is strongly supported by the public'.[24] The wording of this statement suggests that the HFEA had decided, not only that there was a broad public consensus on this issue, but also that the moral reasoning underlying this consensus was convincing.

The exact nature of this reasoning was not clarified in the HFEA's press release. The only indication of the details of the Authority's moral position was given in a letter sent to the Department of Health. In this letter, the reasons offered by 'the public' for rejecting sex selection were listed in terms of the frequency with which they were mentioned in formal replies to the Authority. In descending order of frequency, respondents were said to have expressed concern over the danger of reinforcing sexual stereotypes to the disadvantage of women; the start of a movement down a slippery slope which would end with children being treated as consumer goods; the negative effects that involvement in sex selection would be likely to have on relationships within the family; the probable consequences for the sexual balance of certain ethnic communities; the misuse of medical resources for non-medical purposes; the disturbance of the sexual balance in society as a whole; and the offence caused to God by conduct of this kind.[25] It is unlikely that the Authority endorsed all of these objections to sex selection. It seems reasonable to assume, however, that the HFEA did accept the points made most frequently by respondents about the risk of increased sexual stereotyping and the likelihood of movement down a slippery slope.

What seems to have happened, then, is that, on a modest scale, citizens informed the HFEA that they disapproved of sex selection for non-medical purposes because it would probably reinforce discrimination against women and would eventually undermine some of the values thought to be essential to normal family life. It appears that the HFEA accepted this reasoning and decided without delay to forbid all centres licensed under the 1990 Act from employing sex selection techniques for social reasons.[26] In dealing with this first major issue, the Authority exercised its power in a relatively conservative fashion to limit the application of science-based techniques of assisted reproduction. The HFEA acted promptly, in line with respondents' comments on sex selection, to prevent the products of embryo research from being used in a way that might change the culture of family life or that might strengthen the existing imbalance in relationships between men and women. This seems to provide some confirmation of the argument put forward by the pro-research lobby during the parliamentary debate that the social impact of embryo research would be strictly controlled by the statutory licensing agency.

It does not follow, however, that the HFEA intends to regulate assisted reproduction by introducing a series of rigid rules which confine clinical practice in accordance with the initial public response to each new infertility technique. The Authority stated unambiguously that its decision on sex selection was to be regarded as provisional and that it might be altered in the future in the light of new technical developments or changes in public opinion.[27] Thus, it seems that the HFEA's policy is to exercise control over the products of embryo research in a firm, but at the same time responsive, manner. Although the Authority will ban the use of techniques that are judged to be socially disruptive, it will also keep a regular check on changes in people's attitudes so that, if and when opinions become more favourable, the HFEA will be ready to review the situation and, if appropriate, to give permission for adoption of techniques previously forbidden.

This flexible approach to the application of new developments in reproductive technology is combined with strong support by the Authority for the continuation of embryo research itself, even in areas where there is widespread public opposition and concern. In its control of the research from which the new techniques of assisted reproduction derive, the HFEA seems to be less inclined to pay heed to the views of ordinary people and more determined, if necessary, to act contrary to their wishes. This can be seen clearly in the case of the Authority's decision to authorize the use of reproductive material taken from fetuses and from cadavers for purposes of research.

In both of the HFEA's first two annual reports there was brief reference to the fact that researchers and clinicians had begun to discuss the possibility of using eggs and ovarian tissue from aborted female fetuses, and from other female corpses, for purposes of assisted reproduction. In the second document, published in July 1993, it was stated that the HFEA had no authority to regulate research in this field – presumably because research on human ovaries and eggs did not necessarily involve the creation of human embryos. Nevertheless, it was acknowledged that the Authority did have an interest in research of this kind and a public consultation document was promised which would examine how far, and in what ways, fetal and cadaveric eggs and ovarian tissue might be used for purposes of treatment and research.[28]

In the last week of 1993, there was great excitement in the media over the birth of twins by a British post-menopausal woman and over the request by a black client at Bourn Hall Clinic for implantation of an egg from a white donor. In the first week of 1994, *The Times* extended the discussion of the social tensions arising from assisted reproduction with an article reporting that doctors wanted to use eggs from aborted fetuses in order to help infertile women. The tone of the presentation was critical, with references to 'womb robbing' and 'creating babies from the dead'. In reaction to the article, 'specialists, church leaders, and politicians queue[d] up to express their horror at this proposed treatment, stating that it defies "natural" limits of life and death in reproductive medicine'.[29] The HFEA speeded up the production of its public document on this topic and distributed it widely within a few days. It was noted in the text that 'the emergence of new techniques to alleviate infertility often causes controversy, partly because news of them tends to be broken unexpectedly, sometimes sensationally, to a public unprepared for the issues'.[30]

The consultation document informed its readers that the infertility services in Britain were suffering from a severe shortage of eggs. As a result, research efforts were hampered and many women were forced to wait a long time for treatment. It was explained that there was little chance of increasing the supply of eggs from ordinary, fertile women and that it was, therefore, necessary to consider other potential sources. The two candidates were aborted fetuses, and the bodies of women and girls who had died.[31] The document emphasized that research on donated fetal and cadaveric tissue had been carried out for many years; and that donated organs from corpses and tissue from fetuses were regularly used for therapeutic purposes. Thus the only issue to be decided was whether it was acceptable to use donated *ovarian* tissue, including eggs, from cadavers and aborted fetuses.[32] Although the proposals considered in the consultation document were depicted as being no more than a minor extension of existing practice, it was accepted by the Authority that they raised new ethical issues which needed to be widely discussed and carefully resolved.[33]

By the time that the consultation document was distributed, the HFEA had come to accept that it did have a responsibility for monitoring and regulating scientific research involving fetal and cadaveric eggs as well as clinical treatment using biological material of this kind. It was noted that the capacity to grow and mature human eggs from fetal ovarian tissue was 'still some way off'[34] and that changes in clinical practice would occur, if at all, only after a sustained programme of research. The document, therefore, invited comments on whether eggs or ovarian tissue from cadavers or from aborted fetuses should be used either in research or in treatment.[35]

As in the document on sex selection, the Authority provided a summary of arguments for and against the proposals under consideration. But, in this case, the ethical assessment was heavily biased towards the issue of 'informed consent'. Thirteen out of forty-three paragraphs were devoted to exploring how consent could be properly obtained if the Authority were to grant permission for the use of ovarian tissue and eggs. In contrast, there were only four paragraphs dealing with the broader, and more fundamental, social and ethical issues. These latter paragraphs drew attention to the potential effects on IVF children of knowing that they were born from a fetal or cadaveric egg; to the possible effect of the proposed techniques on the frequency of abortion; to the need to control the number of children born from one donor; and to the existence of widespread doubts about the morality of creating offspring from genetic mothers who had never been born.[36] Although the consultation document's treatment of basic moral issues was brief, the document ended with the statement that the Authority intended to establish a coherent ethical framework for the medical use of human ovarian tissue and eggs.[37]

The document on fetal and cadaveric eggs was distributed much more widely than that on sex selection. Twenty-five thousand copies were dispatched by the Authority and over nine thousand replies were received. The nature of the response, however, was much the same; that is, most people who commented in the media and most of those who replied directly to the HFEA were opposed to the new developments. LIFE organized petitions and a large-scale campaign to persuade people to write to the Authority expressing their disapproval. In Parliament, Dame Jill Knight, acting with the support of the anti-abortion movement, introduced an amendment to the Government's Criminal Justice and Public Order Bill which was designed to 'prohibit the use of eggs from aborted girl babies'[38] in the course of infertility treatment. In her speech, she made clear that she was as much concerned with scientific research in this field as she was with unwelcome changes in clinical practice: 'I want to send a message to scientists that there is no point spending any more time on research in that area, or in messing about with aborted mouse eggs, rat eggs or anything similar. The end product from using aborted human eggs for fertilization purposes will simply not be allowed to be used.'[39]

This amendment, although it was eventually withdrawn, was closely in line with the responses received by the Authority. In its formal appraisal of the results of the public consultation, the HFEA reported that 58 per cent of respondents had condemned the use of fetal eggs for research and 83 per cent had condemned the use of fetal eggs in infertility treatment. Only 7 per cent had actually approved the use of fetal eggs in research and only 3 per cent in treatment. Disapproval of the use of eggs from cadavers was considerable, but more muted. Once again, respondents were more likely to be opposed to the use of such eggs in treatment than in research.[40] The views of the 10,000 individuals who had signed petitions were disregarded on the grounds that they were objecting to abortion rather than to the specific proposals under consideration by the Authority.[41]

The HFEA presented its decisions on this topic in a formal document in July 1994. The Authority noted that there was a 'widespread and fundamental objection' among the general public to the use of fetal ovarian tissue in infertility treatment.[42] It seemed to follow that these negative social attitudes would produce major difficulties for any children born as a result of techniques involving the use of fetal eggs. It was decided, therefore, that no licences for techniques of this kind could be granted by the Authority as long as such attitudes remained dominant. In relation to the use of eggs from adult female corpses for infertility treatment, the Authority stated that it had 'no objection in principle'.[43] But it was decided that the Authority would 'not currently approve its use' because there was considerable uncertainty about the 'psychological consequences for the recipient couple and particularly for the prospective child'.[44] In other words, as in the case of fetal eggs, approval was withheld because of the possible impact of negative social attitudes on those receiving treatment and on those born as a result of treatment. However, in view of the fact that there appeared to be less repugnance at the use of reproductive material from adult corpses in infertility treatment, the Authority proposed to reconsider the matter when more was known about the consequences that might follow from the introduction of cadaveric eggs into clinical practice.

The HFEA's earlier decision with respect to sex selection for social reasons was a genuine restriction on clinical activities because the relevant techniques were already in use for medical purposes. In contrast, the decision on the use of fetal eggs produced a prohibition with no real content. This was so because the development of effective clinical techniques involving such eggs was generally agreed to be some years away. This latter point was made emphatically by a leading medical researcher in a debate in the House of Lords: 'In fact, fertility treatment in adult women using fetal ovarian tissue is not going on, no one is contemplating it, and, even if they were, such a possibility would not be likely to arise for a minimum of 10 to 20 years from the present date.'[45] Thus, although the restraint on clinical practice introduced by the HFEA on the use of fetal eggs was consistent with the bulk of public opinion, it was no more than a formality. The techniques in question were not yet available and could not have been used even if the Authority had given permission. Furthermore, if they were to become available at some future date, the existing ban, formulated in the light of present-day public opinion, would no longer be relevant and the matter would have to be decided afresh on the basis of further consultation.

The crucial decision taken by the HFEA at the end of this period of consultation was not that on treatment, but that on research. The Authority could have banned research on fetal ovarian tissue and, thereby, brought to a stop any further development of clinical techniques. A decision of this kind would have been widely welcomed. As we saw above, the prevention of research was one of the aims behind the actions of the anti-abortion movement. Furthermore, the public consultation had seemed to show that, although people were more concerned about treatment than about research, there was nevertheless considerable anxiety about the latter. The HFEA, however, ignored both the demands of the anti-abortion movement and the opinions of most of its other respondents and declared that donated eggs and ovarian tissue from fetal, as well as from adult, corpses could be used under licence for purposes of scientific inquiry.[46]

The moral reasoning behind the Authority's decision to prohibit treatment, but to permit research, in this area was not made fully explicit in the final report. Despite the promise in the consultation document, no attempt was made in the report to provide a formal statement of the moral framework within which the Authority had reached its conclusions. It is possible to infer from the wording of the text that the HFEA's conclusions, both on treatment and research, were generated by 'balancing benefits against the risk of harm'.[47] This phrase suggests a crude ethical formula which may lie behind the Authority's resolutions. But it does not clarify the crucial issue of how the risks and potential benefits of treatment and research were calculated.

In the case of treatment, some guidance is provided by the statement that 'it would be particularly difficult for a child to come to terms with being produced from a fetus because of prevailing social attitudes'.[48] It appears from this statement that the social disapproval and personal disgust that children born from fetal eggs might experience today, if the techniques in question were in use, were treated as probable costs to be balanced against the possible benefits that might become available when techniques involving fetal eggs have actually been perfected. The implicit reasoning here is confusing, partly because it seems to employ a rather odd comparison between imaginary costs today and possible future benefits. But, given its self-appointed task of judging the morality of infertility treatments that were some way off by reference to their probable consequences, the Authority had no alternative but to try to guess what those consequences might be. Such an approach was bound to be uncertain and subject to unknown errors. However, the Authority may have tried to allow for such errors by basing its conclusions regarding treatment on the conservative assumption that, whenever the techniques under consideration do become available, most people will still find them repugnant and that, as a result, the costs of implementation will remain high.

The HFEA's prohibition of the use of fetal and cadaveric eggs in infertility treatment appears to have been based on a cautious assessment of the probable balance between costs and benefits. The reasoning behind the decision about research clearly involved a more positive estimate of the cost/benefit ratio. Unfortunately, the official report says very little that helps us to understand how the probable consequences of research were assessed. One possibility is that the HFEA, in judging the costs of research on fetal and cadaveric eggs, only considered its *immediate* consequences. If this were so, it may have been assumed that research, unlike treatment, generates no morally relevant costs because it does not produce children who will suffer the unpleasant results of prevailing social attitudes.

Alternatively, it may have been assumed, as the chairman of the HFEA seemed to suggest in a statement to the press, that the views of the general public on this issue were largely irrelevant because few ordinary people properly understood the potential benefits of such research.[49] It may also have been assumed that, once the potential benefits of research became more widely known, public attitudes would begin to change.[50] If such assumptions *were* employed in reaching the decision on research, it is difficult to see why they were not also employed in assessing treatment. For the benefits of research will only become available after the laboratory findings have actually been applied in clinical practice. The lack of clear moral argument in the HFEA's report on this topic means that we cannot know which particular set of assumptions was at work in official reasoning about the morality of scientific investigation. We can be sure, however, that, in one way or another, the cultural impediments that led to the prohibition of treatment were seen as applying less forcefully in the case of research.

The two examples that have been examined in this section show that the HFEA has tried to exercise a restraining influence on the introduction of new clinical practices within the infertility services. It has tried to ensure that infertility treatment does not run ahead of public attitudes and it has tried to take account of those attitudes in assessing the consequences of its own decisions. But, so far as we can judge from these examples, its control of research is likely to be much less restrictive. This may be inevitable. After all, embryo research was approved by Parliament essentially because it was seen to be a potential source of important medical benefits. The Authority is clearly determined to ensure that the scientific community under its guidance is allowed to produce these benefits. However, this asymmetry in the Authority's procedures of ethical control will tend to create further cultural tensions and a growing pressure towards social change. The reason for this is that, whereas the restraints placed by the Authority upon new clinical practices can always be reversed in the light of subsequent events, each decision in favour of a new line of research will tend to produce an irreversible extension in the range of technical possibilities. The examples above suggest that the public will normally respond initially in a negative manner to these new developments. It seems likely, therefore, that, at least in the near future, continuation of the HFEA's current policy will continually generate new areas of social conflict as ordinary people react against a stream of science-based advances in reproductive techniques which challenge their ideas about proper social relationships and normal reproductive conduct.[51]

In the parliamentary debates of the 1980s, the dominant metaphor was that of the 'slippery slope'.[52] Opponents of embryo research repeatedly insisted that the formation of a statutory licensing authority would do very little to prevent further movement down this slope. Its supporters, in contrast, maintained that such an authority would be able to exercise more or less complete control over the progress of research and over its social impact. In the words of Lady Warnock:

I think your Lordships should not be frightened of the slippery slope argument . . . We can stop our descent down the slippery slope at any point when we wish to do so and the way of stopping ourselves descending into unknown horrors is by legislation . . . My belief is that if we have a statutory body licensing research and if the statutory body is backed up by a clear moral view of the pre-embryo, then we need not fear that we shall descend the slope . . . [53]

The developments that have occurred since the establishment of the HFEA will be taken by many to have confirmed Lady Warnock's reassuring prediction. Such people will refer to the fact that the Authority has taken note of public opinion and has restricted the use of currently unacceptable techniques. They will see the policy of regular review of existing restrictions as a reasonable response to the possibility that social attitudes in this area may gradually alter. On the other hand, many people will regard the policy of regular review as a strategy for promoting the slow dissolution of long-standing moral values in the scramble for supposed medical benefits. Such people will regard the decision to ignore public opinion about the use of fetal eggs for purposes of research, and to allow such research to proceed without restriction, as clear evidence that movement down the slippery slope has already begun to accelerate. All concerned are now likely to accept that a cumulative process of technical innovation and cultural change is under way. They will continue to differ, however, in their moral assessment of this process, and they will continue to look into the future with contrasting emotions of hope and of fear.

Social control in Britain and the USA

In the course of the British debate over embryo research, scientists employed a potent image of a future society in which reproductive science would provide a regular supply of technically efficient solutions to a range of medically defined problems. The social ramifications of these technical developments were given little consideration. Scientists were content to leave it to other people to sort out the consequences of introducing their technical achievements into a complex social environment in which participants were committed to values and personal relationships linked to traditional forms of reproduction.

The creation of a statutory licensing authority was recommended in the

Warnock Report as a mechanism for ensuring that the social and moral concerns of non-scientists were properly addressed. In due course, the HFEA was established to reconcile the technical perspective of the scientists with the social and moral requirements of the wider population. In this arrangement, scientists' primary obligations are to improve the existing techniques of assisted reproduction and to furnish new forms of reproductive choice. The external agency is required to monitor and control the development of research, under guidance from representatives of the scientific community; and to moderate the pace at which technical advances are introduced, under guidance from its lay members and from the general public. We saw in the previous section that the HFEA has promoted public discussion of the problems arising from assisted reproduction and that it has adopted a conservative policy of clinical restraint, more or less in line with the cautious optimism of the parliamentary decision in favour of embryo research. It seems likely that most of the cultural tensions that will continue to occur in this area will be resolved slowly and gradually without serious social confrontation or dramatic alterations in reproductive conduct.

In the light of this conclusion, it is worth considering recent developments in the USA, where there has been no sustained public debate on this issue and no national legislation. During the 1980s the Republican administrations of Ronald Reagan and George Bush, under pressure from the pro-life lobby, made sure that no federal funds were available for embryo research.[54] As a result, research of this kind was almost entirely restricted to the private sector, where it was closely tied to the production of commercially viable techniques and profitable clinical practices. In the early 1990s this situation was reviewed by Andrew Kimbrell, who came to the conclusion that the science-based technology of assisted reproduction in the USA was on the verge of running out of control. In the following passage, Kimbrell begins by referring to the research on sex selection carried out by Robert Winston and his colleagues:

While Hammersmith's use of sex selection was designed to prevent disease, the techniques could just as easily be used for simple sex selection. In the future, increasing numbers of couples may undergo IVF and genetic screening of the resulting embryos in order to be implanted only with the embryo that is the sex they desire . . . If parents will screen babies for one nonmedical condition, that is, gender, there is no reason to assume they will not screen them for others. By the next century, many scientists expect that the information gained through the Human Genome Project will enable doctors to screen fetuses and test-tube embryos for an extraordinary variety of physical and behavior traits . . . For the first time in history, parents could be deciding, not wondering, what kind of children they will bear and discarding those seen as imperfect or defective . . . Even with the current limited number of tests for genetic diseases, there is tremendous pressure on doctors and federal agencies to begin massive screening programs that funnel billions of dollars into new biotech screening companies . . . Under pressure from the genetic screening and medical industries, couples in the future may increasingly pick in vitro fertilization rather than natural childbirth . . . Parents could literally pick and choose which embryos have the characteristics that match their desires and discard the others.[55]

This account of the growth of embryo research and assisted reproduction in the USA presents a picture of increasingly rapid changes in reproductive conduct which have been set in motion by major advances in scientific knowledge and technique, combined with unscrupulous commercial manipulation of a credulous public. Kimbrell's predictions are similar to the 'slippery slope' arguments used in the British parliamentary debates and in response to the HFEA's consultation documents. In Britain, such concerns were taken into consideration in the decision to establish the HFEA and in the Authority's own decision to prevent the screening of IVF embryos for purely social reasons. In the USA, in contrast, as Kimbrell notes, there is no legal mechanism to regulate the activities of those engaged either in embryo research or in clinical practice. His disturbing projection of current trends is based on the assumption that this legal vacuum will continue.[56]

In my view, it is unlikely that the new reproductive technologies will have quite such a drastic social impact in the USA as Kimbrell anticipates. In the first place, although there is no external control over embryo research or assisted reproduction, these activities are subject to continual ethical appraisal by the American medical profession.[57] One would expect that some of the innovations in human reproduction envisaged by Kimbrell would be strongly resisted by many members of that profession. Furthermore, if the success rate of IVF does not improve significantly, and there is at present no sign of this happening, it will be technically impossible for parents confidently to pick and choose their children's characteristics in the way that Kimbrell suggests. Thus, reproductive-technology companies will have the difficult task of trying to sell a costly service which frequently fails to deliver.[58] Nevertheless, although his predictions are unlikely to be entirely accurate, Kimbrell does provide a reasonable and well-documented account of the way in which embryo research and assisted reproduction appear to be developing in settings, such as the USA, where commercial interests are powerful and legal restraints are weak.

The situation in the USA has begun to change since Kimbrell published his analysis. In 1993, the Clinton administration abolished the bureaucratic requirement that had prevented government funding of embryo research during the 1980s.[59] Early in 1994, the National Institutes of Health (NIH) responded by setting up the Human Embryo Research Panel to examine whether such research should receive government funds and, if so, under what conditions.[60] The members of the panel were subject to considerable pressure from anti-abortionists.[61] Nonetheless, they decided within the year that research involving human IVF embryos should be eligible for government support under conditions similar to those adopted in the UK. For example, it was proposed that, as in Britain, embryos could be used for research up to the appearance of the primitive streak.[62] Similarly, the panel recommended that certain extreme forms of intervention in the development of IVF embryos should be forbidden, such as cloning by nuclear transfer. In addition, it was proposed that careful consideration should be given to the potentially adverse social consequences of research as well as to 'public sensitivities on highly controversial research proposals'.[63] Despite the restrictions on embryo research recommended by the panel, the NIH was immediately flooded with grant applications from researchers wanting to work in this area.[64]

In broad outline, as well as in many of its details, the proposed framework for control of embryo research in the USA is very much like that in operation in Britain. There is the same conception of the early embryo as a living entity which can be exploited for the common good.[65] There is the same recognition that embryo research may give rise to cultural tensions and to significant changes in social conduct; and the same commitment, in principle, to taking note of these factors in guiding the development of scientific inquiry. There is also a tendency in the report of the Human Embryo Research Panel, as there has been in some of the decisions of the HFEA, to take scientists' claims about potential benefits on trust and to see no need for careful assessment of the moral significance of such benefits.

[The panel] is utterly silent on how research claims and possibilities should be evaluated for their moral weight and benefit. It is no less silent on how, even with that information in hand, a moral calculus is to be constructed to do the necessary balancing... What a free ride this is for the researchers, whose claims of potential benefits are treated with the kind of credulity not seen since the days when the golden calf was worshipped.[66]

If the NIH proposals were to be implemented, it seems likely that the same kind of uncritical estimation of the benefits of embryo research that has begun to appear in the British system of regulation would also tend to occur in the American context. As a result, there would be the same accumulation of science-based technical developments leading to growing pressure for their use in practice. In the USA, however, this pressure would be much stronger and much more difficult to hold in check. The reason for this is that the NIH would have no power over commercial research on human embryos; no capacity to decide what should happen in the infertility clinics; and no control over the use of government-funded results for purposes not anticipated or specified by the researchers. The regulatory procedures put forward by the NIH, unlike those in Britain, would apply only in part of the total system and would have no direct impact on the way in which either new or existing techniques of assisted reproduction were actually used: 'The manipulation of embryos for profit falls outside the authority of NIH embryo guidelines even though the prospects of doing harm and violating social mores may be even greater in the commercial sector than in institutions subject to NIH guidelines.'[67]

It now seems probable that the NIH proposals will not be put into effect without considerable alteration, if at all.[68] President Clinton has made clear that he will not approve the use of human embryos created specifically for purposes of research.[69] Liberal opinion, both in the House of Representatives and in the Senate, is sharply divided over the experimental use of spare embryos, while the powerful pro-life lobby is firmly opposed to embryo research of any kind.[70] The situation resembles the moral and political stalemate that occurred in Britain during the mid-1980s. But the balance of power and the legislative process are quite different in the USA. It is, therefore, impossible to foresee whether any firm decision will ensue or whether the NIH proposals will simply be abandoned. One thing, however, is clear; namely, that a failure to act, and to act in a manner that regulates clinical practice as well as embryo research, will leave the way open for the kind of rapid and disruptive commercialization of human reproduction that was predicted by Kimbrell.

Last words and future prospects

The debate over embryo research in Britain involved a clash between two contrasting images of the future. The scientists promised a future in which, due to their efforts, childlessness would be less prevalent than ever before and the horrors of genetic disease would be steadily reduced. Their opponents saw a future in which traditional family values would be undermined and existing social relationships seriously damaged by the unanticipated consequences of scientists' pursuit of reproductive control. The majority of decision-makers in Parliament shared many of these fears about the potentially disturbing social impact of embryo research. But they were unwilling to give up the major benefits promised by the research community. As a result, they voted for the establishment of a system of social control which was intended to help bring the scientists' vision into being, whilst preventing the unwanted side-effects envisaged by their opponents.

The regulative body that emerged from the embryo debate looks constantly into the future in order to try to estimate potential benefits and costs, and to make morally informed decisions about scientific research and its practical application. As a result of these decisions, a new world of human reproduction is slowly being established. In this world, the moral boundaries that define the limits of research will gradually be revised, in a piecemeal fashion, as scientists repeatedly press for permission to explore newly discovered therapeutic possibilities. Similarly, the moral boundaries that restrict the clinical use of reproductive science will also change as science-based techniques extend the range of reproductive possibilities and as people come to accept that human reproduction has no set form. Although the degree of technical control over reproductive processes will increase, each step forward will reveal new problems that will be seen as requiring further scientific inquiry and new kinds of technical intervention. There will, however, be no mad rush down a slippery slope. Rather, in Britain, there will be cautious, gradual, almost imperceptible movement into a future in which nothing will be certain except that, in the long run, the practices, expectations, values and morality associated with human reproduction will have been transformed.

Epilogue:

Intruders in the fallopian tube or a dream of perfect human reproduction

I was on my way home to Clapham yesterday evening and, as I got off the bus, I saw this newspaper placard: **ONE MILLIONTH TEST-TUBE BABY**. I was shocked. Could it be that many already? After all, the first successful *in vitro* fertilization was as recent as 1978. Surely, I thought, this is typical exaggeration by the media. However, on reflection, I realized that there must now be many thousands of test-tube babies around. After all, there are fifty or so IVF clinics operating in France alone, over forty in Britain and a great many more throughout the other advanced nations. Sooner or later, therefore, even if this particular newspaper report is wrong, that figure of one million will eventually be reached.

Perhaps I had better explain before I go any further how I come to know this kind of detail about the spread of IVF. The fact is (it's still difficult to say it in a straightforward way), my husband and I are unable to have children. This condition is not unusual, I assure you. About one in ten couples are infertile for one reason or another. So when Dr Edwards developed the IVF technique and began to help childless people to have kids, I read everything I could on the subject. Unfortunately, we were too old to try for a test-tube baby ourselves; and anyway we didn't have enough money. But I became very interested in people's reactions to IVF and to the research on human embryos that Dr Edwards and other scientists have to carry out in order to make it work properly.

When I first heard about IVF, my own reaction was simple. It seemed to me that there were lots of couples who wanted a baby but were physically unable to produce one; that a technique was now available which sometimes, but not always, led to successful pregnancy for such people; and that further research was needed on human embryos in order to make the technique more reliable. However, as I followed the debate that occurred during the 1980s, I became aware that not everybody saw it my way. Indeed, some of them seemed to think that basic moral principles were being infringed and that no further research should be allowed at all. Even Dr Edwards and his colleagues, I was surprised to find, called for moral guidance from the wider society.

That 'wider society', of course, includes people like me. But the more I have examined the issues, the more confused I have become. There seem to be so many conflicting points of view, each of which is entirely convincing on its own, yet which lead to very different courses of action regarding IVF and embryo research. Over the years, I have come to believe that it's quite impossible to devise a single policy that is consistent with the full range of opinions on this topic to be found in British society. Nevertheless, an official policy did eventually emerge, which is taken to express some vague national consensus, and an executive body for licensing embryo research has been established which puts this policy into operation.

Internationally, the situation is even more chaotic. Even a pretence of consensus is impossible. For instance, in France, IVF is a thriving business, yet there is a voluntary moratorium on some of the critical lines of related research. In Germany, all such research is forbidden. In Italy, there are no restrictions on research, even though the Catholic Church is fundamentally opposed to its continuation. Research is possible in the United States, but federal agencies will not provide any money for it. And in Australia, the situation varies from one state to another. In other words, both within and between the first world countries, the response to embryo research has been extremely varied; and the overall situation is remarkably confused.

Well, all of this, and much more, went through my mind yesterday evening after I reached home and told my husband about the headline. It seemed to us, as we talked it over, that the whole affair arose from the difficulties involved in trying to take control over the processes of human reproduction. We were particularly struck by the way that improvements in technical control had unexpected repercussions in the realm of social control. For instance, the researchers and the doctors, in order to help people like us, had developed these new medical techniques which were designed to make controlled reproduction possible in those cases where it didn't occur naturally. But this gave rise to moral choices which, in turn, had to be controlled by agreed ethical principles. So, in those countries where embryo research wasn't forbidden, the researchers had to be subject to morally informed regulation; and organizations had to be set up to carry out this regulation. However, these official agencies themselves had to be controlled; that is, they had to be seen to operate in a way that was morally acceptable to most, although not necessarily all, of the members of their particular society. Thus, improvements in technical control created a need for moral control, which required organizational and legal control to implement the moral decisions, which depended, in turn, on the exercise of political and social control. I don't think I've expressed that very clearly. But I hope you see what I mean.

When these questions first began to be explored during the early 1980s, the 'great British public', on the whole, seemed to be very much against the IVF enterprise. Or rather, they liked people having babies, but they seemed not to like the research that made the babies possible. However, scientists and doctors in Britain worked hard to explain what was really involved in embryo research and to show that there was nothing wrong with it. At the same time, 'pro-lifers' and others who had moral qualms tried equally strenuously to argue against it. The outcome was a typical British compromise; that is, that officially licensed research was to be allowed, but only during the first fourteen days of an embryo's existence. After that, these minute creatures were to be 'allowed to die' because, when they reached this age, it would be immoral to use them for research. Any scientist caught handling an embryo more than fourteen days old (excluding any time spent by the embryo in a frozen state) would be subject to criminal charges.

This arrangement came to be widely applauded in the UK as an exemplary solution, and it was thought that many other nations would eventually see its wisdom and sort their problems out in a similar fashion. But I had never been convinced that this arrangement was going to work in the long run and, as I prepared for bed, I wondered whether the British approach was an adequate response to the complex debate I had observed during the preceding decade.

THE DREAM

I am sitting at a raised table. Stretching away from me is a tunnel which curves out of sight to the left. The roof is low and I feel narrowly confined. Thin filaments reach out from the pitted surface of the tunnel and waft gently in the warm current. In the distance is a steady, low throbbing. From around the curve I can hear an irregular soft plopping, like the sound of ripe follicles budding. At a short distance, there is a seething crowd of simple life forms. One of them seems to react to my presence and comes towards me in a slow and awkard, yet clearly purposeful, fashion. Despite its primitive level of organic structure, it begins to speak.

FIRST LIFE FORM In order to decide what to do about research on human
    embryos, we need to know what human embryos are. Once we have
    clarified what they are, it will be fairly obvious how we should treat

them. Let us consider the biologically simplest, and therefore morally the most extreme, case of the one-cell human zygote, conceptus or embryo. It is evident that such a creature is living biological material. This is true, but unhelpful. For it doesn't distinguish the early form of the human embryo from a vast range of other biological stuff in relation to which, it is generally agreed, moral considerations do not arise. We could try to be more specific, in order to find the locus of the moral issues associated with research on human embryos, and describe the zygote as 'human genetic material'. But again the phrase is too indiscriminate and would cover human genes, chromosomes or a segment of DNA. We can, in practice, identify the essential meaning of 'human embryo or conceptus' only by drawing attention to its potential for maturing, under the right conditions, into an individual human being.

A human embryo, even in its most basic form, is therefore distinguished by being a living member of the species *homo sapiens*. One might respond to this claim by pointing out that the zygote has a long way to go before it becomes a fully developed human person and that its moral status, therefore, must be in various ways less than that of a mature person. But this observation is confused. It fails to separate the contingent practical fact that there are a limited number of moral issues that arise in people's dealings with embryos from the more fundamental question of the embryo's moral standing. Although moral relationships with embryos are restricted by the simplicity of their present organic structure, their moral status is determined by their capacity to become fully developed human beings and to enter, in due course, into the human community. The abilities of human adults are only explicable if the inherent capacity for those abilities was always present in the crude organisms from which such adults matured. It is this potential for achieving a particular type of development that is significant in deciding what kind of being an embryo is. It follows that human embryos are to be treated morally according to the same principles as other individual human persons, for they contain within them the same essential human capacity.

In recognizing the equality of status of all members of the human family, we are led to adopt the principle of equality of respect for all human persons. This means that our essential respect for human individuals must be absolute and cannot be traded off against supposedly beneficial outcomes which may follow from a possible course of action. Thus human persons, including embryos, cannot justifiably be treated as someone else's property. Human persons, including embryos, cannot ethically be used as a means for someone else's gain, whether financial, medical or otherwise. We have no alternative but to conclude that human embryos, even in their earliest form as one-cell zygotes, cannot be used as experimental material without immorally disregarding their humanity. We must, therefore, prohibit research on human embryos; no matter how well intentioned the scientists involved and irrespective of any increase they may promise in their ability to satisfy the needs or desires of adult human beings.

[As this speech draws, in measured periods, to its conclusion, another life form moves alongside the initial speaker. This second creature approaches rapidly, its long tail darting sharply from side to side, and is already in mid-utterance when it comes within earshot. Its statements overlap with and intersect the first monologue.]

SECOND LIFE FORM . . . is a continuous process passed on from one generation to the next. All forms of life, whether humans, animals or plants, are fundamentally alike. Human reproduction is not essentially different from that of other animals. The same organs, structures, hormones and molecules are involved.

When human fertilization occurs, the egg and sperm merge to form a single cell. Contrary to common belief, however, the two pronuclei donated by the male and female do not fuse together within this single cell. Thus a clearly defined moment indicating that fertilization has occurred cannot be identified. It makes no biological sense to regard fertilization as a point in time from which each individual's origin can be unequivocally traced.

It should also be noted that the single-cell zygoyte is totipotential; that is, from it develop not only all the different types of tissues and organs that make up the human body, but also the tissues that become the placenta and fetal membranes in the course of intra-uterine development. In other words, at this early stage there is no biological distinction between those elements that will become the biological organism and those that will be naturally discarded as the waste products of reproduction. This totipotential capacity is retained, to some extent, throughout the first developmental phase of the human embryo so that, if particular cells are separated, each cell may proceed to form its own independent embryo. During the early stages of embryonic growth, human cells are undifferentiated. Until they have become further organized and until they have become implanted in a human womb, they do not constitute a biological individual, still less a person with rights or other moral attributes.

Individual human life, then, does not begin at fertilization but later. The cells that are destined to form the embryo itself do not appear in humans before about day five. When the true embryo first starts to develop, some fourteen or fifteen days after fertilization, it still has no differentiated tissues or organs and no nervous system. It is doubtful whether there are any convincing grounds for treating this emergent creature as a human person; but there is room here perhaps for differences of judgment. It is, however, absolutely clear that the four- or eight-cell organism that is used in *in vitro* fertilization and in the so-called 'embryo transfer' procedure is actually a functionally undifferentiated preimplantation embryo which is in no way a human being.

Once we understand the biological facts, it becomes evident that the moral rules governing our treatment of other human actors are irrelevant to research on human embryos. Thus there are no moral considerations that need prevent us from pursuing the major medical benefits that such research can produce. As everybody knows, significant advances in the treatment of infertility have already been achieved by scientists working on early embryos. But it is important to stress that, in due course, research of this kind will enable us to understand, detect and control many, perhaps most, forms of congenital disease. It will also lead to reductions in the frequency of miscarriage and, almost certainly, in the development of new techniques of contraception. Finally, we should not forget that research on human embryos is itself in its early stages of growth and that, as it moves towards maturity, we may expect that benefits as yet undreamed of will flow from the inventiveness and creativity of the scientists who are active in this field.

In conclusion, let me say that I do not wish to deny that values and morality enter into this area of scientific activity. But we should not be misled into a vain projection of human characteristics upon unfeeling biological processes. Rather, our endeavours must be guided by the hopes of living men and women for children of their own; children who are free from the tragic effects of genetic or chromosomal abnormality. Our moral commitment must be, not a fearful defence of the status quo, but the vigorous and hopeful pursuit of a better world.

[At this point, two more life forms join the jostling nucleus which is beginning to accumulate around me. One of them responds to the contrasting arguments put forward so far.]

THIRD LIFE FORM Finding a consensus with regard to an embryo's legal–ethical right to protection is made all the more difficult because opinion on this matter is often prejudiced by the desire to give the researcher either more or less freedom of action. Those who wish to encourage research on embryos tend to deny their human quality from the start. They base their arguments on the lack of individual personality in the pre-nidation phase or simply on the fact that abortion is not illegal at that phase. Those who, on the contrary, find abortion as well as embryo research indefensible, believe their position already established by assuming that the embryo, from the time of fertilization, has the individuality and personality of a human being and thus is entitled to its own basic legal rights.

Neither of these extreme positions is satisfactory. For instance, even if the embryo has human qualities, it is no more entitled to freedom from all interference than is an individual who has been born. Even the right to life is contingent upon circumstance; as in time of war, when individuals may be required to sacrifice their lives for what is officially deemed to be the greater good of the community. Thus, the use of relative standards in deciding about the protection of unborn life does not appear to be inconceivable.

On the other hand, it would be just as incorrect to conclude that the embryo is not a person or does not have a right to protection simply because abortion is not a criminal offence. Very wisely, the criminal code avoids any definition of human life and limits itself to describing the boundaries of criminal liability. In order to regulate the conduct of research on human embryos, we do not need to decide when 'personhood' commences. For we are by definition dealing with life that originates from human germ cells and is in this sense different from any other plant or animal life, not to speak of mere things. Thus we can hardly deny all moral status to these entities which have the potential to become human beings.

My view, therefore, is that we should abandon any attempt to try to settle, once and for all, the ontological standing of the human embryo; and that we should concentrate instead on the practical task of specifying the degree to which and the circumstances under which new human entities can be manipulated and, indeed, destroyed in order to bring about beneficial outcomes. There are clearly three different sets of circumstances to be considered. When the expected research results can benefit the particular embryo being studied, we are dealing with a therapeutic trial for which appropriate guidelines are already available. A second situation arises when the research is intended to benefit other embryos or other persons, but not the embryos under study. In such cases, the death of the subject embryos may be justified only if this result is unavoidable and if the use of these embryos is outweighed by the potential medical gains. Finally, there is the situation where embryos are directly and solely produced for research purposes. In this context, the destruction of human life is planned at the same time as its creation. Such lack of concern for human dignity is difficult to justify, no matter what the intended goal, for it involves a fundamental estrangement and instrumentalization of human existence.

This is, of course, but a first sketch of how we must begin to chart a middle course through these difficult problems. I believe that it is . . .

[The third speaker is here interrupted by the other life form in whose company it had arrived.]

FOURTH LIFE FORM . . . necessary to stand back and adopt a broader, more socially informed, perspective. One fundamental limitation to so much of the discussion is that it takes the new technology of human reproduction as an independent variable and proceeds to examine the range of possible ethical and legal responses that might be adopted in order to restrict its consequences. The basic error in such an approach is that it fails to recognize that the technology is itself a social product which is intimately bound up with other social factors and that these social factors extend well beyond the confines of the scientific or the medical communities.

For example, it is clear that the new reproductive technology emerged at a time when the traditional solution to the problem of infertility, that is, adoption, was becoming less effective owing to changing patterns of contraception, the wider availability of legal abortion, and changing attitudes to the one-parent family. In other words, there were less babies around for adoption by infertile couples. The personal pressures to which Steptoe and Edwards reacted in their pursuit of IVF and the test-tube baby were not accidental. They were the predictable outcome of large-scale changes in the patterns of conduct in modern industrial societies which had made particular cases of infertility more difficult to resolve.

Social influences on the emergence of IVF can also be seen in the way that the scientists' definition of the problem they were addressing was formed in accordance with the ideas of proper family life dominant in their culture, and in line with a uniquely modern notion of the purpose of medical intervention. Thus the new technology of human reproduction was designed on the assumption, for instance, that family membership should be a matter of controlled parental choice rather than, for example, a haphazard by-product of sexual activity or a consequence of God's inscrutable decision. At the same time, the technology took for granted that medicine was no longer confined to remedying disease and disability, but should take an active role in helping people to realize their thwarted desires. Social, or cultural, assumptions such as these do not merely provide the context in which technologies operate. They are, rather, intrinsic to the sets of ideas through which technologies, including that of IVF and its associated practices, acquire their particular shape.

The fact that technologies are part of the fabric of society and that assumptions about social relationships enter into the design of technologies does not mean, however, that the introduction of new technologies necessarily proceeds smoothly and without unanticipated social repercussions. Indeed, unexpected consequences almost always occur. This is partly because new technologies themselves tend to change and develop rather quickly, so that initial ideas about implementation soon become outdated. But it is also because, in modern societies, the wider social context is complex, differentiated and itself undergoing continual alteration. As a result, the responses to new technologies are often varied and to some degree unforeseen.

We can observe this clearly in the case of IVF. For example, although IVF was partly a response to the changing pattern of family life in the 1960s and 1970s, its first practical application was as a technique for helping people who were unable to have a conventional nuclear family. Consequently, many of the unanticipated moral problems arising from its use have emerged as people have tried to employ IVF and associated techniques to extend the range of new and unconventional family structures. Thus the possibilities of 'rent-a-womb', 'virgin' mothers, homosexual 'families', or the selective use of 'high-quality sperm', were not acknowledged, and probably not envisaged, on the day that Louise Brown was born in Oldham to two very ordinary parents. Nevertheless, these possibilities were implicit from the start in the broader social context where personal life, among certain sectors of society, was coming to be flexibly and individually fashioned in accordance with members' increasingly variable desires.

If we wish to understand, and to control, the impact of new technologies, we need to think of them as emergent forms of social action embedded within larger and diverse social settings. We must, of course, pay proper attention to what we are told about such technologies by the scientists, by the moralists and by the legal experts. But their relatively narrow, disciplinary perspectives, taken alone or in conjunction, will never enable us to construct effective management strategies. For none of them takes us to the transformative social dynamic that generates and moulds technologies and gives them meaning. It follows, therefore, that we will eventually have to respond to the challenge of human reproductive technology with a greatly increased programme of research into the social processes of technological change. Only in this way will we be able to ensure that its uses are kept within acceptable limits. If this is not done, society will be forced into an unending series of unstable ethical compromises as the technology develops and is exploited in new ways by a variety of culturally discrepant groups.

My message, then, in its most general form, is that the growing commitment by modern societies to biological technology will inevitably require a major commitment to the techniques of social engineering. Furthermore, given that the biological technology of the future will necessarily become widely available within the industrial nations, I am led to conclude that social control will have to be implemented on an international basis. Thus the ethical debate concerning the moral status of the person has actually focused on a derivative issue. The more fundamental issue is that of the proper balance between individual control and centralized control of people's personal lives. I have no doubt that a greater degree of centralized control will be found to be more consistent with the maintenance of social order.

[As this speech unfolds, its tone becomes increasingly portentous and I begin to find it somewhat disturbing. I look around to see how the others are reacting and I am surprised to find that the number of life forms clustered about my desk has doubled without my noticing. Several of them seem to be keen to speak, but they conform to some unstated order of precedence and all but one remain quiet.]

LIFE FORM FIVE The explicit formulation of defensible moral principles and the creation of social agencies for their implementation is specially characteristic of modern times. The reasons for this are fairly obvious. One important factor is the diffusion of scientific thought throughout many areas of social life together with the fact that the resulting technical advances have increasingly generated novel problems to which traditional moral precepts are not easily applied. In addition, modern societies tend to be pluralistic, in the cultural as well as the social-structural sense of this term. This means that different ideologies compete for the individual's allegiance and provide a range of diverse resources which are available in relation to each new problematic situation.

It is rarely the case that a social group can fully articulate its moral stance, even in connection with a very specific and well-defined set of social activities, or provide clear justification for its moral position in a way that is persuasive for those who do not belong to that group. In traditional societies, where there is considerable moral consensus and where the legitimacy of established practices remains largely taken for granted, the tacit and incomplete character of moral belief seldom gives rise to major difficulties. In the modern world, however, it can lead to incomprehension of others' views and bitter confrontation as contradictory moral solutions are advanced and defended. Such moral polemics are likely to become particularly difficult to resolve when those involved in the debate claim to speak for some third party which has no voice of its own and which cannot, therefore, comment on or arbitrate concerning the claims made on its behalf. It is evident that the debate over embryo research and the moral status of embryos is of this kind.

One of the essential features, then, of the embryo debate is that participants are dealing, among other things, with the standing of possible moral agents who are themselves unable to take part in the debate. The linguistic incapacity of the embryo is of fundamental importance because it may be argued that the ability to participate in human discourse is a defining characteristic of a moral agent and, indeed, of a person. Thus rights may be attributed to non-speakers such as animals or embryos. But the attribution of rights can only be carried out by actors capable of formulating them; and the responsibility to fulfil rights can be applicable only to actors able to understand the requirements of a moral code. Insofar as being a person is the same as being a moral agent, it seems to follow that embryos, fetuses and, I must add, very young children are not persons.

In the light of these considerations, it is not surprising that, when we examine the embryo debate carefully, we find that the frequent use of the term 'person' is quite misleading. For even those arguing in defence of the embryo's humanity and personhood actually claim only that the embryo has the potential eventually to become a person. Thus there is an implicit recognition that the development of the person requires entry into a linguistic community and, as a consequence, that the central issue in relation to the continuation of embryo research is something other than personhood. In practice, the debate hinges around different assessments of the point at which the individual biological organism can be discerned. Those who are against research tend to choose the 'moment of fertilization', whilst those in favour tend to select the emergence of the 'primitive streak' or some later transition in the sequence of biological development. It is evident that these choices do not specify the appearance of the human person; they deal rather with the appearance of that type of organism that can, in principle, become the biological locus of personhood.

If the embryo debate is not really about personhood, we need an alternative description which will capture its essential character. I suggest that it is fruitful to see this moral confrontation as a power struggle among different sectors of modern society concerning the boundary between the human and the non-human. Both sides of the dispute agree that we are morally obliged to be relatively restrained when we intervene in the human domain. Both sides also agree that less stringent moral standards govern mankind's use of the non-human and that the non-human is, therefore, more fully open to exploitation in pursuit of human interests. What separates the opposing camps is that they draw the boundary around humanity either more or less widely. Those arguing for a ban on research include more of the biological world within the human province; whilst those advocating research draw the line more narrowly, thereby extending the range of human manipulation.

In order to win a struggle of this kind in a modern society, the opposing parties must attract a sufficient level of support from the uninformed and initially uninterested mass of the population. The great strength of the conservative, 'pro-embryo' or 'anti-research' party is that it can convincingly claim to embody traditional values and to be resisting the insidious immorality of the present-day world. However, its main weakness lies in its inability to offer any tangible gain. Adherence to its ideology may confer a sense of moral probity, but no practical benefits. Indeed, those against embryo research often find themselves having to acknowledge that their position may imply a considerable degree of sacrifice, not only on their own part, but also on the part of society at large. In contrast, those in favour of research base their case heavily on the practical improvements already achieved and, even more, on the promise of significant advances yet to come. Thus, in terms of classical moral categories, a division has emerged between those defending basic human rights and those advocating the application of a utilitarian calculus of benefits.

The first practical success of the science of human reproduction was to make human birth possible where previously it had been impossible. This achievement alone, however, did not produce wide public agreement about the need to continue research in this field. One reason may well have been that the gain in human fertility was of personal interest to no more than a minority of people. In addition, infertility tended to rank relatively low in the priority list of conditions requiring medical treatment. For it was neither life-threatening nor physically disabling. The decisive swing in favour of the science lobby did not occur, therefore, until the late 1980s, when scientists began to link embryo research to the conquest of genetic defects and diseases. This change in rhetorical emphasis was probably critical in mobilizing support for embryo research because the fear of conceiving a congenitally defective child is widespread, if not universal, among human beings. Reproductive science held out, for the first time, the possibility of removing this threat – if not for the parents of today, perhaps for their children or their children's children.

Scientists were, thus, able to achieve an initial victory in the struggle over the continuation of embryo research at least partly by claiming that they would be able, in due course, not only to provide children for almost everybody who wanted them, but also to ensure that virtually all children would be born without significant defects. As a result of the moral confrontation arising out the creation of IVF, certain scientists, claiming to speak on behalf of the research community, have been led to promise effective control over both the occurrence and the quality of human reproduction. Where this will lead them and us is not yet clear. It is certain, nevertheless, that their intellectual and technical journey will sooner or later call for major moral adjustments, even transformations of moral perspective, from ordinary people such as ourselves.

[At this point, an illuminated slide is suddenly projected against the wall of the tunnel. It shows a dense mass of penguins which fill the frame in their thousands. I am at first confused. What has this got to do with the speaker's story about a cultural power-struggle? Are we to be given the point of view of these non-humans? But then I realize that the slide belongs to the next contributor.]

LIFE FORM SIX Take a good look at those penguins and observe the uniformity of phenotype. This lack of variation is the result of the strong pressure of natural selection under conditions of limited survival chances. Now look at these slides showing the enormous range of variation among domesticated animals and among human beings. From these observations, we can safely conclude that humans have long been able to manipulate the genetic constitution of many species, including their own genome. In this respect, the introduction of the new reproductive technologies is simply an extension of well-established practices. All that has changed in recent years is that control has begun to be linked more firmly and directly to the findings of systematic scientific experiment.

Control over human reproduction is being transferred steadily from society at large to the research community. There is no turning back from this process. For scientific knowledge and techniques are necessarily superior to the resources for exercising control that are otherwise available. Furthermore, the first full-scale scientific revolution in human reproduction, arising out of the critical encounter between *in vitro* reproduction and genetics, has already passed beyond the planning stage. The initial concern of this revolution is the genetic diagnosis of IVF embryos before transplantation for couples that are known to carry genetic anomalies. It is now beginning to become possible for man, not merely to tinker with the surface features of his own reproduction as in the past, but to master the quality of his progeny. We already know in principle how to achieve this goal. In due course, knowledge of this kind must inevitably lead to dramatic changes in our reproductive practices.

There are more than three thousand known genetic abnormalities in humans and at least one of them is present in around 1 per cent of all live births. The percentage of human carriers is, of course, considerably higher than this. The combination of IVF and genetic analysis will enable us to identify diseases such as cystic fibrosis, Duchenne muscular dystrophy, thalassaemia, sickle-cell anaemia, Down's syndrome, Huntington's disease, phenylketonuria, and many others, at an early stage in the embryos' development and to replace in the womb only those that are free of these conditions. Given time and enough resources, we will be able to eliminate most, perhaps all, of these terrible diseases. We are certain that this can be done. It would be immoral not to make sure that it *is* done.

The modern world is confronted with the fact that research is paving the way for choice of future children according to qualities that will have been specified in advance. Can we stop when we have complete control over genetic disease? Should we even try to stop there? Surely the answer to both those questions is 'No!' Science-based medicine is no longer concerned solely with disease but, more fundamentally, with removing unnecessary barriers to the realization of our desires. Partial restrictions, bans and moratoria may well be placed on the research that will make possible the satisfaction of these desires. But once we have the basic knowledge, or even know that such knowledge is possi-

ble, it will prove futile to try to maintain a policy of deliberate ignorance. We have no genuine alternative, therefore, but to commit ourselves to constructing in the real world mankind's perennial dream of
perfect reproduction.

[Oh dear, will they never cease talking! There seem to be more of them than
ever. I'm surrounded now by a great cloud of throbbing life forms. I hope
they don't all want to have their say. I'll never get out of here. I wish I could
just close my eyes and go to sleep.]

LIFE FORM SEVEN Akan tetapi jika kita menekankan ciri kontinjen secara
budaya tentang ilmu pengetahuan sains itu . . . (the speech of life form
seven fades into the background and is replaced by a voice-over) . . .
your way of living in the world is so strange. Your pursuit of personal
goals is so unswerving. Yet you lack any true idea of the person with
which to guide your steps. I fear for you and I fear even more for your
children.

Every human life is a process of becoming in the world. Some of you
are half aware of this. Traces of the old wisdom remain. But it is
strangely altered by your systems of thought, by your science and your
social science, by your law and your morality. In looking so closely at
the parts of the world, you have lost sight of the whole.

Each of us is given life by the ancestors and each of us returns to the
ancestors when the time comes. The completed person is the product
of a whole life. The value of that life can be judged in full only by the
ancestors. We cannot know that judgment. Nevertheless, we do know
that it is based, not on the extent of our devotion to the self, but on the
way in which we have given sustenance to the other.

We become persons by fulfilling our obligations to the other. This
includes our family, our neighbours and our ancestors. But also
included are those other-than-humans who make up the wider world
of our being and whose ancestors gave birth to our ancestors. A true
human person does not seek ever greater control over the other, but
rather listens to the voice of the other and measures its needs against
the needs of the other.

The person is finally realized in death. Death is to be welcomed and
embraced as the gateway to the realm of the ancestors. In your world,
death is deeply feared. Yet death is also denied. Once you have taken
control of life and are able to produce it at will, you will turn to death
and strive to remove it from your world. Perfect human specimens
living forever . . . walaupun begitu, kami tidaklah bercadang melan-
jutkan isu yang komplaks ini dengan lebih jaun lagi . . .

VOICES OFF

Come and look at this one.

Have you done the gene amplification?

Yes. It's clearly pathological.

My goodness, you're right. Five consecutive sentences mentioning death.

That means the text is morbid, doesn't it?

Yes, it does. This is one of the worst cases of cultural nostalgia I've ever seen.

What would happen if we allowed this text to mature?

There can be no doubt that the greater the technological progress to be achieved in years to come, the more this text would yearn for some vague, unattainable state of tribal innocence.

So, it would be grossly maladapted to modern society.

Yes, that's right. There's only one possible course of action.

To the shredder?

To the shredder!

Notes

Introduction

1 Robert Edwards and Patrick Steptoe, *A Matter of Life: The Story of a Medical Breakthrough* (London: Hutchinson, 1980).

2 Gena Corea, *The Mother Machine: Reproductive Technologies from Artificial Insemination to Artificial Wombs* (London: The Women's Press, 1985), p. 119.

3 Human Fertilization and Embryology Authority, *Annual Report* (London: HFEA, 1992), p. 9.

4 Andrew Kimbrell, *The Human Body Shop: The Engineering and Marketing of Life* (San Francisco and London: HarperCollins, 1993), p. 88.

5 Michael Mulkay, *The Social Process of Innovation* (Basingstoke: Macmillan, 1972).

6 Edward Yoxen, 'Conflicting concerns: the political context of recent embryo research policy in Britain', in M. McNeil, I. Varcoe and S. Yearley (eds.), *The New Reproductive Technologies* (Basingstoke and London: Macmillan, 1990), pp. 173–99.

7 Michael Mulkay, 'Changing minds about embryo research', *Public Understanding of Science* 3 (1994), 195–213.

8 Derek Morgan and Robert G. Lee, *Human Fertilization and Embryology Act 1990: Abortion and Embryo Research, the New Law* (London: Blackstone, 1991).

9 The Warnock Report on Human Fertilization and Embryology contains a five-page appendix listing those organizations and individuals who provided evidence for the Committee. It is mentioned that, in addition, 695 letters and submissions were received from the public. See Mary Warnock, *A Question of Life: The Warnock Report on Human Fertilization and Embryology* (Oxford: Blackwell, 1985), pp. 99–105.

10 Morgan and Lee, *Human Fertilization and Embryology Act 1990*, note 8, chapters 3–4; HFEA, *Annual Report* (1992), note 3.

11 Warnock, *A Question of Life*, note 9, p. vi.

12 Ibid., p. iii; for a clear summary of the Warnock proposals, see Jennifer Gunning and Veronica English, *Human In Vitro Fertilization: A Case Study in the Regulation of Medical Innovation* (Aldershot: Dartmouth, 1993), pp. 36–41.

171

13 Michael Mulkay, 'Embryos in the news', *Public Understanding of Science* 3 (1994), 33–51.

14 The main debates used in this study are as follows: *Parliamentary Debates* (Hansard), **House of Lords:** Fifth Series, Human Fertilization: Warnock Report, vol. 456, 31 October 1984, cols. 524–93; Human Fertilization and Embryology, vol. 491, 15 January 1988, cols. 1450–1508; Unborn Children (Protection) Bill, vol. 504, 8 March 1989, cols. 1538–80; Human Fertilization and Embryology Bill, vol. 513, 7 December 1989, cols. 1002–114; Human Fertilization and Embryology Bill, vol. 515, 8 February 1990, cols. 950–90: **House of Commons:** Sixth Series, Human Fertilization and Embryology (Warnock Report), vol. 68, 23 November 1984, cols. 547–90; Unborn Children (Protection) Bill, vol. 73, 15 February 1985, cols. 637–98; Human Fertilization and Embryology, vol. 126, 4 February 1988, cols. 1202–61; Human Fertilization and Embryology Bill, vol. 170, 2 April 1990, cols. 914–90; Human Fertilization and Embryology Bill, vol. 171, 23 April 1990, cols. 31–133. At certain points, reference is also made to the following shorter parliamentary sessions in the House of Commons: Unborn Children (Protection) Bill, vol. 74, 3 May 1985, cols. 576–95; Unborn Children (Protection) Bill, vol. 74, 7 June 1985, cols. 612–15; Unborn Children (Protection) (No. 2) Bill, vol. 102, 21 October 1986, cols. 971–7 (London: HMSO).

15 All items dealing with research on human embryos were extracted from *New Scientist* (eighty-five items) and from the news section of *Nature* (seventy-nine items) between 1984 and 1990.

16 Items on embryo research were extracted systematically from all the British national newspapers and from the leading provincial papers from the end of November 1989 to the beginning of July 1990 by Lincoln Hannah (Mediascan) Ltd. The total number of items is 218. This includes only those items that focused on embryo research and/or the technologies of assisted reproduction such as IVF. It does not include press cuttings dealing mainly with the clause on abortion that was added to the Human Fertilization and Embryology Bill and which was widely discussed in the newspapers. Of these 218 cuttings, 133 consist of direct reports about parliamentary debate.

17 The following official reports were consulted in the course of this study: *Report of the Committee of Inquiry into Human Fertilization and Embryology* (London: HMSO, 1984); Department of Health and Social Security, *Legislation on Human Fertility Services and Embryo Research: A Consultation Paper* (London: HMSO, 1986); *Human Fertilization and Embryology: A Framework for Legislation* (London: HMSO, 1987); Jonathan Glover et al., *Fertility and the Family: The Glover Report on Reproductive Technologies to the European Commission* (London: Fourth Estate, 1989); *Human Artificial Procreation* (Strasbourg: Council of Europe, 1989); The Interim Licensing Authority, *IVF Research in the UK 1985–89* (London: ILA, 1989); The Interim Licensing Authority, *Statistical Analysis of the United Kingdom IVF and GIFT Data 1985–90* (London: ILA, 1990); Jennifer Gunning, *Human IVF, Embryo*

Research, Fetal Tissue for Research and Treatment, and Abortion: International Information (London: HMSO, 1990); *Report of the Committee on the Ethics of Gene Therapy* (London: HMSO, 1992); Human Fertilization and Embryology Authority, *Annual Report* (London: HFEA, 1992, 1993, 1994).

18 The following studies of embryo research, IVF and related topics have been consulted in carrying out this study: Corea, *The Mother Machine*, note 2; Kimbrell, *The Human Body Shop*, note 4; Yoxen, 'Conflicting concerns', note 6; Morgan and Lee, *Human Fertilization and Embryology Act*, note 8; Gunning and English, *Human In Vitro Fertilization*, note 12; Jeanette Edwards, Sarah Franklin, Eric Hirsch, Frances Price and Marilyn Strathern, *Technologies of Procreation: Kinship in the Age of Assisted Reproduction* (Manchester: Manchester University Press, 1993); Marilyn Strathern, *Reproducing the Future; Essays on Anthropology, Kinship and the New Reproductive Technologies* (Manchester: Manchester University Press, 1992); Jose Van Dyck, *Manufacturing Babies and Public Consent: Debating the New Reproductive Technologies* (Basingstoke: Macmillan, 1995); Patricia Spallone, *Beyond Conception: The New Politics of Reproduction* (Basingstoke: Macmillan, 1989); Lynda Birke, Susan Himmelweit and Gail Vines, *Tommorow's Child: Reproductive Technologies in the 90s* (London: Virago, 1990); Meg Stacey (ed.), *Changing Human Reproduction: Social Science Perspectives* (London: Sage, 1992); Dorothy Nelkin, *Selling Science: How the Press Covers Science and Technology* (New York: W. H. Freeman, 1987); Ruth Hubbard, *The Politics of Women's Biology* (New Brunswick: Rutgers University Press, 1990); Patricia Spallone, *Generation Games: Genetic Engineering and the Future for Our Lives* (London: The Women's Press, 1992); McNeil, Varcoe and Yearley (eds.) *The New Reproductive Technologies*, note 6; Brian Bloomfield and Theo Vurdubakis, 'Disrupted boundaries: new reproductive technologies and the language of anxiety and expectation', *Social Studies of Science* 25 (1995), 533–51; Irma van der Ploeg, 'Hermaphrodite patients: in vitro fertilization and the transformation of male infertility', *Science, Technology and Human Values* 20 (1995), 460–81. For discussion of the need for inquiry into the wider political and cultural context of scientific development, see Susan E. Cozzens and Thomas Gieryn (eds.), *Theories of Science and Society* (Bloomington: Indiana University Press, 1990); Andrew Pickering, *The Mangle of Practice: Time, Agency and Science* (Chicago: Chicago University Press, 1995); and Michael Gibbons et al., *The New Production of Knowledge: The Dynamics of Science and Research in Contemporary Society* (London: Sage, 1994). For discussion of the relationship between human bodies and technology, see Donna J. Haraway, *Simians, Cyborgs, and Women: The Reinvention of Nature* (London: Free Association Books, 1991); and Stuart Blume, *Insight and Industry: On the Dynamics of Technological Change in Medicine* (Boston: MIT Press, 1992).

1 The background to the debate

1 Peter G. Richards, *Parliament and Conscience* (London: Allen & Unwin, 1976).

2 Richards, *Parliament and Conscience*, note 1; Madeleine Simms, 'Legal abortion in Great Britain', in Hilary Homans (ed.), *The Sexual Politics of Reproduction* (Aldershot: Gower, 1985), pp. 78–95.

3 Richards, *Parliament and Conscience*, note 1, chapter 9; Keith Hindell and Madeleine Simms, *Abortion Law Reformed* (London: Peter Owen, 1971), pp. 165 and 201.

4 Richards, *Parliament and Conscience*, note 1, p. 111; Hindell and Simms, *Abortion Law Reformed*, note 3, p. 201; Simms, 'Legal abortion in Great Britain', note 2, pp. 80–3. The Abortion Bill was introduced by a young Liberal MP who happened to have been placed high in the ballot for Private Member's legislation. But the Bill would not have been enacted without active help from the Labour Home Secretary or without the votes of a large proportion of the Labour membership of the House.

5 Richards, *Parliament and Conscience*, note 1, pp. 108–9.

6 Simms, 'Legal abortion in Great Britain', note 2, pp. 90–5.

7 Hindell and Simms, *Abortion Law Reformed*, note 3, p. 16.

8 Ibid., p. 87.

9 Ibid., p. 82.

10 Ibid., p. 16.

11 Ibid., p. 112.

12 Simms, 'Legal abortion in Great Britain', note 2, p. 84.

13 *Social Trends* 15 (1985), 44.

14 Robert Edwards and Patrick Steptoe, *A Matter of Life: The Story of a Medical Breakthrough* (London: Hutchinson, 1980), p. 82.

15 Henry Leese, *Human Reproduction and In Vitro Fertilization* (London and Basingstoke: Macmillan, 1988), p. 32.

16 Edwards and Steptoe, *A Matter of Life*, note 14; Leese, *Human Reproduction*, note 15; John D. Biggers, 'Pioneering mammalian embryo culture', in B. D. Bavister (ed.), *The Mammalian Preimplantation Embryo* (New York: Plenum Press, 1987), pp. 1–22; Gena Corea, *The Mother Machine: Reproductive Technologies from Artificial Insemination to Artificial Wombs* (London: The Women's Press, 1985).

17 Edwards and Steptoe, *A Matter of Life*, note 14, p. 102.

18 *Social Trends* 10 (1980), chart 2.21; Alexina M. McWhinnie, 'Test-tube babies . . . the child, the family and society', in S. Fishel and E. M. Symonds (eds.), *In Vitro Fertilization: Past, Present, Future* (Oxford: IRL Press, 1986), pp. 215–27.

19 *Social Trends* 10 (1980), 90.

20 Hindell and Simms, *Abortion Law Reformed*, note 3, p. 30.

21 In strict terms, adoption deals with the problem of childlessness, but leaves the condition of infertility unchanged. The same can be said of IVF. Nevertheless, both IVF and adoption enable some infertile people to have children. In this practical sense, they can be regarded as at least partial solutions to some of the emotional and social problems caused by infertility.

22 Lesley Rimmer and Malcolm Wicks, 'The family today', in Eric Butterworth and David Weir (eds.), *The New Sociology of Modern Britain* (London: Fontana, 1984), pp. 33–9.

23 Miriam David, 'Moral and maternal: the family and the Right', in Ruth Levitas (ed.), *The Ideology of the New Right* (Cambridge: Polity Press, 1986), p. 140.

24 Rimmer and Wicks, 'The family today', note 22; McWhinnie, 'Test-tube babies', note 18.

25 McWhinnie, 'Test-tube babies', note 18; Corea, *The Mother Machine*, note 16, pp. 146–8; Leese, *Human Reproduction*, note 15, p. 32. The relevance of male infertility has also come slowly to be recognized. See Lynda Birke, Susan Himmelweit and Gail Vines, *Tomorrow's Child: Reproductive Technologies in the 90s* (London: Virago, 1990), pp. 88–90. More recently, the possibility of a decline in male fertility as a result of the presence of quasi-oestrogens in the environment has begun to receive attention: 'Assault on the male', *Horizon*, BBC 2, 11 April 1994.

26 For an excellent discussion of this topic, and related issues, see Jose Van Dyck, *Manufacturing Babies and Public Consent: Debating the New Reproductive Technologies* (Basingstoke: Macmillan, 1995), chapter 3; see also Birke, Himmelweit and Vines, *Tomorrow's Child*, note 25, pp. 65–7.

27 Malcolm Potts and Peter Selman, *Society and Fertility* (Plymouth: Macdonald & Evans, 1979), pp. 83 and 249–55. Despite all the discussion of the supposed increase in infertility among women in recent decades, it seems clear that, if we count demographically enforced childlessness outside marriage as well as involuntary infertility within marriage, the overall rate of female infertility has actually declined since the 1960s. The increase in childlessness among women has been confined to the married population. The reduction in socially enforced childlessness has passed unnoticed. It is likely, however, that the increasingly widespread use of IVF will lead to attempts to define other kinds of socially marginal childlessness as legitimate infertility.

28 Edwards and Steptoe, *A Matter of Life*, note 14, p. 119. Implantation of fertilized human ova began in 1971.

29 Ibid., pp. 101–2.

30 Jennifer Gunning and Veronica English, *Human In Vitro Fertilization: A Case Study in the Regulation of Medical Innovation* (Aldershot: Dartmouth, 1993), p. 6; Edward Yoxen, 'Conflicting concerns: the political context of recent embryo research policy in Great Britain', in M. McNeil, I. Varcoe and S. Yearley (eds.), *The New Reproductive Technologies* (Basingstoke and London: Macmillan, 1990), pp. 173–99, at p. 180.

31. Edwards and Steptoe, *A Matter of Life*, note 14, p. 84.

32 Ibid., p. 113.

33 Robert Edwards, *Life before Birth: Reflections on the Embryo Debate* (London: Hutchinson, 1989), chapter 1.

34 R. G. Edwards, 'Test-tube babies, 1981', *Nature* 293 (24 September 1981), 253–6. The medical community helped to increase demand for assisted reproduction by

broadening the definition of infertility and by drawing attention away from the high failure rates. See Van Dyck, *Manufacturing Babies*, note 26, chapter 3.

35 In practice, both success rates and access to IVF were very slow to increase. See Corea, *The Mother Machine*, note 16, pp. 179–80; Birke, Himmelweit and Vines, *Tomorrow's Child*, note 25, pp. 122–4 and 126–7. The link between the pro-abortion case and the moral argument for embryo research was stated clearly in *New Scientist* several years later where it was argued that infertile women have as much right to bear children as fertile women have not to bear them; and that if science can help such women, it has a duty to do so: 'Embryonic Arguments', *New Scientist* 105 (14 February 1985), 2.

36 Edwards and Steptoe received a standing ovation at a crowded meeting of the Royal College of Obstetricians and Gynaecologists in January 1979. See Edwards and Steptoe, *A Matter of Life*, note 14, p. 184; see also Corea, *The Mother Machine*, note 16, p. 116.

37 Edwards and Steptoe, *A Matter of Life*, note 14, p. 187.

38 Ibid., p. 188. For an informed discussion, from the perspective of the early 1980s, of the moral issues likely to arise from embryo research and IVF, see Clifford Grobstein, 'Coming to terms with test-tube babies', *New Scientist* 96 (7 October 1982), 14–17.

39 Richards, *Parliament and Conscience*, note 1, p. 206.

40 Ibid., p. 103.

41. Hindell and Simms, *Abortion Law Reformed*, note 3, pp. 112–21 and 189–90.

42 Richards, *Parliament and Conscience*, note 1, p. 104.

43 Hindell and Simms, *Abortion Law Reformed*, note 3, p. 95.

44 Richards, *Parliament and Conscience*, note 1, p. 109.

45 *LIFE News*, No. 28 (Summer 1995), p. 1. This is a silver jubilee edition of *LIFE News* in which an account is given of the formation of LIFE between May and August 1970.

46 Ibid., p. 1. In addition to providing an efficient 'pro- life pregnancy care service', LIFE has systematically undertaken 'grass-roots pro-life educational work': ibid.

47 Leo Abse, 'The politics of in vitro fertilization in Britain', in S. Fishel and E. M. Symonds (eds.), *In Vitro Fertilization: Past, Present, Future* (Oxford: IRL Press, 1986), pp. 207–13; Simms, 'Legal abortion in Great Britain', note 2. By 1978, LIFE had established 150 groups throughout the UK. By 1980, it had opened its fortieth Care Centre. This number had increased to 120 by 1992. See *LIFE News*, note 45, p. 6.

48 Simms, 'Legal abortion in Great Britain', note 2, p. 91.

49 This was taken by many Catholics to be the official view of the Roman Catholic Church. Thus the Catholic community was very active in opposition to the 1967 Abortion Act. See Hindell and Simms, *Abortion Law Reformed*, note 3, chapter 4. For a careful examination of the Catholic position on abortion, IVF and embryo research, see Kenneth Boyd, Brendan Callaghan and Edward Shotter, *Life before Birth: A Search for Consensus on Abortion and the Treatment of Infertility* (London: SPCK, 1986).

50 This wider view of the significance of the pro-life cause has tended to become more clearly established over time. See *LIFE News*, note 45, p. 4. See also Hindell and Simms, *Abortion Law Reformed*, note 3; Simms, 'Legal abortion in Great Britain', note 2; David, 'Moral and maternal', note 23; Yoxen, 'Conflicting concerns', note 30; Abse, 'The politics of in vitro fertilization in Britain', note 47.

51. David, 'Moral and maternal', note 23; Yoxen, 'Conflicting concerns', note 30. As we saw earlier in this chapter, marriage and conventional family life actually became more frequent at this time. But this change was partly hidden by the cultural invisibility of spinsterhood. It was also obscured statistically by an increase in the proportion of elderly couples with no resident children, in the proportion of elderly people living alone, and by changing patterns of divorce and remarriage. Nevertheless, in accordance with the fears of the moral conservatives, there were genuine increases during the 1960s and 1970s in the frequency of informal cohabitation, in the frequency of conception and birth among the unmarried, and in the frequency of employment of married women outside the home. See McWhinnie, 'Test-tube babies', note 18; Rimmer and Wicks, 'The family today', note 22; and *Social Trends* 15 (1985), 42–3.

52 David, 'Moral and maternal', note 23; Yoxen, 'Conflicting concerns', note 30.

53 David, 'Moral and maternal', note 23; Yoxen, 'Conflicting concerns', note 30.

54 Hindell and Simms, *Abortion Law Reformed*, note 3, p. 102.

55 David, 'Moral and maternal', note 23, p. 161. David's original source is Ronald Butt, 'Not only moral but right', *The Times*, 7 March 1985.

56 Yoxen, 'Conflicting concerns', note 30, p. 184.

57 Ibid.

58 David, 'Moral and maternal', note 23, p. 154.

59 Yoxen, 'Conflicting concerns', note 30, pp. 180–1.

60 Edwards and Steptoe, *A Matter of Life*, note 14, p. 188; see also Grobstein, 'Coming to terms', note 38.

61. Yoxen, 'Conflicting concerns', note 30, pp. 184–8.

62 *Parliamentary Debates* (Hansard) House of Lords, AID and In Vitro Fertilization, vol. 432, 9 July 1982, col. 1001. For full bibliographical details of quotations from Hansard, see note 14 of the Introduction.

63 Mary Warnock, *A Question of Life: The Warnock Report on Human Fertilization and Embryology* (Oxford: Blackwell, 1985). The Warnock Committee was composed of seven scientists and/or doctors, three persons from the legal profession, two social workers, one professor of theology, one director of a charitable trust and one head of a health authority. Warnock was a moral philosopher. At least six members of the Committee were women. Anti- abortionists have frequently complained that their views were not represented on the committee. For a discussion of the operation of the Warnock committee, see Lady Mary Warnock, 'Government commissions', in U. Bertazzoni, P. Fasella, A. Klepsch and P. Lange (eds.), *Human Embryos and Research: Proceedings of the European Bioethics Conference Mainz 1988* (Frankfurt/New York: Campus Verlag, 1990), pp. 159–68.

64 Warnock, *A Question of Life*, note 63, Introduction and pp. 80–6 where the full set of recommendations is listed.
65 Ibid., p. 80.
66 Ibid., p. 8.
67 Ibid., p. 1.
68 Ibid., p. 11.
69 Ibid., p. 10.
70 Ibid., pp. 80–6.
71 The Conservative majority in the Commons over Labour in 1985 was 188. This was even larger than the Labour majority over the Conservatives in 1967 which was 110. See David Butler, *British General Elections since 1945* (Oxford: Blackwell, 1989), Appendix 1.
72 Yoxen, 'Conflicting concerns', note 30, pp. 184–8; Derek Morgan and Robert G. Lee, *Human Fertilization and Embryology Act 1990: Abortion and Embryo Research, the New Law* (London: Blackstone, 1991), pp. 38–9 and 74–7.
73 Sir Bernard Braine, Commons, Human Fertilization and Embryology (Warnock Report), vol. 68, 23 November 1984, cols. 539–44. Sir Bernard regularly spoke on behalf of the SPUC in Parliament.
74 *Warnock Dissected: A Commentary on the Report of the Committee of Inquiry into Human Fertilization and Embryology* (Leamington Spa: LIFE, 1984).
75 Ibid., p. 20.
76 Braine, Commons, 23 November 1984, cols. 539–44.
77 Abse, 'The politics of in vitro fertilization in Britain', note 47, pp. 210–11.
78 Yoxen, 'Conflicting concerns', note 30, p. 183.
79 Edwards, *Life before Birth*, note 33, chapter 5.

2 The sequence of parliamentary debate

1 Edward Yoxen, 'Conflicting concerns: the political context of recent embryo research policy in Great Britain', in M. McNeil, I. Varcoe and S. Yearley (eds.), *The New Reproductive Technologies* (Basingstoke and London: Macmillan, 1990), pp. 173–99.
2 Derek Morgan and Robert G. Lee, *Human Fertilization and Embryology Act 1990: Abortion and Embryo Research, the New Law* (London: Blackstone, 1991).
3 Mary Warnock, *A Question of Life: The Warnock Report on Human Fertilization and Embryology* (Oxford: Blackwell, 1985), pp. 64 and 75.
4 Ibid., p. 64.
5 Omar Sattaur, 'New conceptions threatened by old morality', *New Scientist* 103 (27 September 1984), 12.
6 Ibid.
7 Ibid., 13.
8 'Confused comment on Warnock', *Nature* 312 (29 November 1984), 389.
9 Ibid.

10 Mary Warnock, 'Scientific research must have a moral basis', *New Scientist* 104 (15 November 1984), 36.

11 'Warnock fuels debate over 14-day rule', *New Scientist* 103 (26 July 1984), 3.

12 Warnock, 'Scientific research', note 10, 36.

13 Ibid.

14 Ibid.

15 'Lords oppose embryo research', *New Scientist* 104 (8 November 1984), 6.

16 *Parliamentary Debates* (Hansard), House of Commons, Human Fertilization and Embryology (Warnock Report), vol. 68, 23 November 1984, cols. 551–2. For full bibliographical details of quotations from Hansard, see note 14 of the Introduction.

17 Ibid., cols. 587–8.

18 'Confused comment', note 8, 389.

19 Leo Abse, 'The politics of in vitro fertilization in Britain', in S. Fishel and E. M. Symonds (eds.), *In Vitro Fertilization: Past, Present, Future* (Oxford: IRL Press, 1986), pp. 207–13.

20 Enoch Powell, Commons, 15 February 1985, col. 640.

21 Steve Connor, 'Voluntary controls placed on embryo research', *New Scientist* 105 (24 January 1985), 21; Jennifer Gunning and Veronica English, *Human In Vitro Fertilization: A Case Study in the Regulation of Medical Innovation* (Aldershot: Dartmouth, 1993), pp. 41–3.

22 Connor, 'Voluntary controls', note 21, 21.

23 'Warnock proposals in trouble', *Nature* 313 (7 February 1985), 417.

24 Ibid.

25 Powell, Commons, 15 February 1985, col. 637.

26 Forty-seven per cent of the membership of the Commons voted on this occasion. This is a relatively high level of participation for Private Member's legislation. See Peter G. Richards, *Parliament and Conscience* (London: Allen & Unwin, 1976).

27 Norman St John-Stevas, Commons, 15 February 1985, col. 649.

28 Steve Connor, 'MPs vote to ban embryo research', *New Scientist* 105 (21 February 1985), 3.

29 Ibid.

30 Maxine Clarke, 'British Commons vote for ban', *Nature* 313 (21 February 1985), 618.

31 'An appeal to embryologists', *Nature* 314 (7 March 1985), 11.

32 Ibid.

33 H. John Evans and Anne McLaren, 'Unborn Children (Protection) Bill', *Nature* 314 (14 March 1985), 127–8.

34 Abse, 'The politics of in vitro fertilization', note 19, p. 212.

35 Ibid., p. 213; Unborn Children (Protection) Bill, vol. 74, 3 May 1985, cols. 576–95.

36 Maxine Clarke, 'Government stops Powell Bill', *Nature* 314 (18 April 1985), 573.

37 Maxine Clarke, 'Embryo protection bill resurfaces', *Nature* 315 (13 June 1985), 534; Abse, 'The politics of in vitro fertilization', note 19, p. 213.

38 Steve Connor, 'Scientists licensed to work on pre-embryos', *New Scientist* 108 (21 November 1985), 21; Maxine Clarke, 'Chances of legislation fade', *Nature* 318 (21 November 1985), 197.

39 Connor, 'Scientists licensed to work', note 38, 21; Clarke, 'Chances of legislation', note 38, 197.

40 The Voluntary Licensing Authority had come into operation in June and began to issue licences for research in November. Connor, 'Scientists licensed to work', note 38, 21; Gunning and English, *Human In Vitro Fertilization*, note 21, chapter 4.

41 Clarke, 'Government stops Powell Bill', note 36, 573.

42 William Cash, Commons, Human Embryos, vol. 90, 24 January 1986, col. 555. The signatories acted on behalf of LIFE's membership of 30,000 persons.

43 Ibid.

44 Maxine Clarke, 'Another bill bites the dust', *Nature* 319 (30 January 1986), 349.

45 Ken Hargreaves, Commons, 21 October 1986, cols. 971–3.

46 Peter Thurnham, Commons, 21 October 1986, cols. 973–4.

47 This interpretation would have been modestly strengthened if it had been noted that the rate of participation in the vote had increased from 47 per cent to 55 per cent.

48 Anne McLaren, 'Embryo research', *Nature* 320 (17 April 1986), 570. This item is a letter written by the embryologist on the Warnock Committee in reply to queries raised by a former editor of *Nature* about the term 'pre-embryo': see note 49. For a discussion of the usefulness of the term from the perspective of the VLA, see Gunning and English, *Human In Vitro Fertilization*, note 21, pp. 57–9.

49 David Davies, 'Embryo research', *Nature* 320 (20 March 1986), 208.

50 Edwin Chargaff, 'Engineering a molecular nightmare', *Nature* 327 (21 May 1987), 199–200.

51 'IVF remains in legal limbo', *Nature* 327 (14 May 1987), 87.

52 'Playing with words', *New Scientist* 108 (21 November 1985), 17.

53 *Legislation on Human Infertility Services and Embryo Research* (London: HMSO, 1986), Cm 46.

54 Gail Vines, 'Government seeks views on "test-tube" babies', *New Scientist* 112 (18 December 1986), 3.

55 Ibid.; Peter Newmark, 'UK legislation further delayed', *Nature* 324 (18/25 December 1986), 604.

56 *Human Fertilization and Embryology, a Framework for Legislation* (London: HMSO, 1987), Cm 259.

57 Warnock, *A Question of Life*, note 3, p. 74.

58 *A Framework for Legislation*, note 56, p. 7.

59 Ibid.

60 See, for example, the Earl of Lauderdale, Lords, 15 January 1988, cols. 1485–7. The impression given in Gunning and English's description of events is that the

Department of Health and Social Security was strongly in favour of the Warnock proposals. See *Human In Vitro Fertilization*, note 21, esp. p. 42.

61 'Shattered test tubes', *New Scientist* 116 (3 December 1987), 21; Simon Hadlington, 'British Government hedges bets on embryo research', *Nature* 330 (3 December 1987), 409. See also chapter 8 below.

62 'Britain hazards embryo research', *Nature* 330 (3 December 1987), 407.

63 'Tough talk on surrogate birth', *Nature* 320 (13 March 1986), 95. This statement was made in the course of a discussion of embryo research, IVF and surrogacy.

64 Tam Dalyell, 'Embryos, plutonium and slippery subs', *New Scientist* 117 (17 March 1988), 71.

65 'Britain hazards', note 62, 407.

66 Ibid.; 'Shattered test tubes', note 61, 21.

67 Gail Vines, 'Legislative plans threaten embryo research', *New Scientist* 116 (3 December 1987), 23.

68 Baroness Lane-Fox, Lords, 15 January 1988, col. 1475.

69 'Embryonic arguments against test-tube baby work', *New Scientist* 117 (17 March 1988), 24.

70 Ibid.; 'Shattered test tubes', note 61, 21.

71 Tam Dalyell, 'Forests, embryos and optoelectronics', *New Scientist* 119 (22 September 1988), 69–70.

72 Christine McGourty, 'Pressure on UK for embryo bill', *Nature* 336 (8 December 1988), 505.

73 Ibid.; see also Gunning and English, *Human In Vitro Fertilization*, note 21, p. 88.

74 The Duke of Norfolk, Lords, 8 March 1989, col. 1538.

75 Lord Houghton, Lords, 8 March 1989, col. 1542.

76 Fifteen Members spoke in favour of the Bill and ten Members spoke against.

77 Lord Houghton, Lords, 8 March 1989, col. 1591.

78 'Church leader claims embryo research conflicts with human rights', *New Scientist* 124 (11 November 1989), 22.

79 Ibid.

80 Andy Coghlan, 'Peers set the tone for Commons debate on embryo research', *New Scientist* 125 (17 February 1990), 19.

81 'Decision time for embryo research', *New Scientist* 124 (25 November 1989), 21.

82 Ibid.

83 Tam Dalyell, 'Wrong way to proceed on embryos', *New Scientist* 124 (18 November 1989), 69; 'Campaigners count their fire power', *New Scientist* 124 (25 November 1989), 22.

84 Dalyell, 'Wrong way to proceed', note 83; 'Embryo research and abortion', *Nature* 341 (26 October 1989), 673.

85 Coghlan, 'Peers set the tone', note 80.

86 The Archbishop of York, Lords, 7 December 1989, cols. 1019–22.

87 Lords, 7 December 1989, cols. 1002–14.

88 Lord Prys-Davies, Lords, 7 December 1989, col. 1105.
89 Coghlan, 'Peers set the tone', note 80.
90 Ibid.
91 Tam Dalyell, 'Loans, embryos and trees on the move', *New Scientist* 125 (3 March 1990), 70.
92 Peter Aldhous, 'Pressure stepped up on embryo research', *Nature* 344 (19 April 1990), 691.
93 'Abortion from a hat', *Nature* 344 (5 April 1990), 476.
94 Aldhous, 'Pressure stepped up', note 92.
95 'Abortion from a hat', note 93. *Nature* had argued much earlier that the time-limit for legal abortion should be reduced because the technology for the preservation of fetuses born prematurely had improved in the past twenty-five years, whilst there had also been many improvements of the diagnosis of pregnancy: 'Britain hazards', note 62, 407.
96 'Abortion from a hat', note 93.
97 Morgan and Lee, *Human Fertilization and Embryology Act 1990*, note 2, p. 38.
98 Peter Aldhous, 'Pro-life actions backfire', *Nature* 345 (3 May 1990), 7.
99 'Campaigners count', note 83.
100 Aldhous, 'Pressure stepped up', note 92.
101 Ibid.
102 Jo Richardson, Commons, 23 April 1990, col. 46.
103 Aldhous, 'Pro-life actions', note 98; Andy Coghlan, 'Parliament gives over-whelming approval to embryo research', *New Scientist* 126 (28 April 1990), 29.
104 Tam Dalyell, 'Doom and gloom pays off', *New Scientist* 126 (12 May 1990), 75.
105 Ibid.
106 Aldhous, 'Pro-life actions', note 98.

3 Political parties and ministerial tactics

1 For full bibliographical details of quotations from Hansard, see note 14 of the Introduction: Norman Fowler, Commons, 23 November 1984, cols. 528–33; Kenneth Clarke, Commons, 23 November 1984, col. 587; Lord Glenarthur, Lords, 31 October 1984, col. 525.
2 Lord Skelmersdale, Lords, 15 January 1988, col. 1451.
3 Clarke, Commons, 15 February 1985, cols. 678–9.
4 Tony Newton, Commons, 4 February 1988, col. 1203.
5 Clarke, Commons, 15 February 1985, col. 680.
6 Ibid.
7 In 1985, 304 MPs voted, that is, 47 per cent of the House of Commons. In 1990, 551 MPs voted, that is, 85 per cent of the House of Commons.
8 D. Marsh, P. Gowin and M. Read, 'Private Member's Bills and moral panic: the case of the video recordings bill (1984)', *Parliamentary Affairs* 39 (1986), 179–90.
9 Fowler, Commons, 23 November 1984, col. 528; Clarke, Commons, 2 April 1990, col. 915.

10 Clarke, Commons, 2 April 1990, col. 916.

11 Virginia Bottomley, Commons, 23 April 1990, col. 125.

12 Glenarthur, Lords, 31 October 1984, col. 589.

13 Clarke, Commons, 23 November 1984, cols. 586–90; Clarke, Commons, 15 February 1985, cols. 679–85.

14 Lord Mackay, Lords, 7 December 1989, col. 1008.

15 Ibid.

16 Clarke, Commons, 23 April 1990, col. 40.

17 Clarke, Commons, 15 February 1985, cols. 681–2; Skelmersdale, Lords, 15 January 1988, col. 1450.

18 Fowler, Commons, 23 November 1984, col. 529.

19 Newton, Commons, 4 February 1988, col. 1208.

20 See the speeches cited above. The implicit alliance between Government and the pro-research lobby is also evident in the way in which ministers were persuaded by the representatives of that lobby to depart from customary procedure and to consider the clauses on embryo research first in the Lords, rather than in the Commons. See chapter 2 above. In addition, one of the ministers who became involved in guiding the Government Bill through Parliament had previously been a parliamentary representative for the MRC. See Bottomley, Commons, 4 February 1988, col. 1247 and 2 April 1990, cols. 981–5. Finally, it seems that the Department of Health and Social Security was inclined to favour implementation of the Warnock proposals. See Jennifer Gunning and Veronica English, *Human In Vitro Fertilization: A Case Study in the Regulation of Medical Innovation* (Aldershot: Dartmouth, 1993), chapters 3–4.

21 For example, Alistair Burt, Commons, 23 April 1990, cols. 113–14.

22 Clarke, Commons, 23 November 1984, col. 588.

23 See Fowler, Commons, 23 November 1984, col. 529, where it is stated that Mr Clarke was 'in overall charge of consultation' following the Warnock Report.

24 In their study of the legislative changes concerning abortion in Britain during the 1960s, Hindell and Simms suggest that Government 'neutrality' is often a polite euphemism for positive obstruction or active sympathy: Keith Hindell and Madeleine Simms, *Abortion Law Reformed* (London: Peter Owen, 1971), p. 86. In the present case, Mr Clarke's active sympathy for embryo research is particularly evident. For suggestions by parliamentarians that the Government were waiting for opinion to change, see Ken Hargreaves, Commons, 4 February 1988, col. 1250 and Lord Houghton, Lords, 8 March 1989, col. 1541.

25 Skelmersdale, Lords, 15 January 1988, col. 1504. I think that his Lordship's figures exaggerate the majority in favour of embryo research in this debate.

26 Ibid., col. 1508.

27 In 1985, 192 Conservatives voted on embryo research out of 397. In 1986, 226 Conservatives voted on this topic.

28 P. Norton and A. Aughey, *Conservatives and Conservatism* (London: Temple Smith, 1981).

29 Peter G. Richards, *Parliament and Conscience* (London: Allen & Unwin, 1976), p. 27.
30 Richards, *Parliament and Conscience*, note 29, p. 179. These divisions within the Conservative Party should not be conceived as uniform, stable groupings, but as ideological coalitions with loose and fluctuating memberships. The same is true of the Labour Party.
31 For example, Norton and Aughey, *Conservatives*, note 28; I. Crewe and D. Searing, 'Ideological change in the British Conservative Party', *American Political Science Review* 82 (1988), 361–84; P. Norton, '"The lady's not for turning" but what about the rest? Margaret Thatcher and the Conservative Party', *Parliamentary Affairs* 43 (1990), 41–58.
32 Norton and Aughey, *Conservatives*, note 28, p. 13; see also R. Garner and R. Kelly, *British Political Parties Today* (Manchester: Manchester University Press, 1993).
33 Norton and Aughey, *Conservatives*, note 28, pp. 19–20 and 65.
34 Elizabeth Peacock, Commons, 23 November 1984, cols. 557–9.
35 Michael Mulkay, 'Science and family in the Great Embryo Debate', *Sociology* 28 (1994), 699–715.
36 Norton and Aughey, *Conservatives*, note 28, p. 13.
37 Crewe and Searing, 'Ideological change', note 31, 367.
38 Norton and Aughey, *Conservatives*, note 28, p. 79.
39 Ibid. The progressive movement is represented here more or less in its own terms.
40 Clarke, Commons, 23 April 1990, col. 41.
41 Ibid., col. 42.
42 Baroness Hooper, Lords, 7 December 1989, col. 1111.
43 Douglas Hogg, Commons, 15 February 1985, cols. 697–8.
44 Maxine Clarke, 'Chances of legislation fade', *Nature* 318 (21 November 1985), 197. The Prime Minister's public remarks about embryo research suggest that, on this issue, she accepted the views and recommendations of the scientific authorities. See Peter Thurnham, Commons, 21 October 1986, col. 974, and the Earl of Bessborough, Lords, 7 December 1989, col. 1080. In this respect, she did not differ from the leaders of the other major parties who also supported, and voted for, the continuation of licensed embryo research. Mrs Thatcher differed from most members of her own party, however, in openly adopting this position very early in the sequence of debates.
45 Three members of Cabinet voted for Powell's Bill, one voted against (the Secretary of State for Social Services), and fourteen abstained. The Minister for Health was not a member of Cabinet. These figures and those given in the main text refer to parliamentarians who had seats in the Commons.
46 Clarke, Commons, 15 February 1985, col. 687.
47 David Butler, *British General Elections since 1945* (Oxford: Blackwell, 1989).
48 *Report of the Annual Conference of the Labour Party, 1985*, p. 129.
49 Garner and Kelly, *British Political Parties*, note 32, p. 71.
50 H. M. Drucker, *Doctrine and Ethos in the Labour Party* (London: Allen &

Unwin, 1979). There are, of course, divisions within the Labour Party as well as within the Conservative Party. In the Labour Party, however, these divisions arise out of different views concerning the way in which the move towards a more egalitarian society should be accomplished. See E. Shaw, *Discipline and Discord in the Labour Party* (Manchester: Manchester University Press, 1988).

51 Harry Cohen, Commons, 23 November 1984, cols. 572–3.

52 Leo Abse, 'The politics of in vitro fertilization in Britain', in S. Fishel and E. M. Symonds (eds.), *In Vitro Fertilization: Past, Present, Future* (Oxford: IRL Press, 1986), pp. 207–13.

53 Forty-eight per cent of Conservatives (192) and 41 per cent of Labour MPs (86) voted on this occasion.

54 See D. N. Campbell-Savours, Commons, 15 February 1985, cols. 658–9; Dr J. Bray, Commons, 15 February 1985, cols. 691–2. Religious affiliation may have been a significant consideration for some of those opposed to embryo research in both parties. But religion was also widely used to justify support for such research. Its influence on the debate was far from straightforward. See chapter 7 below.

55 Commons, 3 May 1985, cols. 592–3.

56 Abse, 'The politics of in vitro fertilization', note 52, p. 213. The impact of the 'New Right' or the 'Moral Right' on the reaction to embryo research and the new technology of assisted reproduction is discussed in M. Durham, 'Family, morality and the New Right', *Parliamentary Affairs* 38 (1985) 180–91; Miriam David, 'Moral and maternal: the family and the Right', in Ruth Levitas (ed.), *The Ideology of the New Right* (Cambridge: Polity Press, 1986), pp. 136–68; Edward Yoxen, 'Conflicting concerns: the political context of recent embryo research policy in Great Britain', in M. McNeil, I. Varcoe and S. Yearley (eds.), *The New Reproductive Technologies* (Basingstoke and London: Macmillan, 1990), pp. 173–99.

57 *Report of the Annual Conference of the Labour Party, 1985*, p. 100.

58 Ibid., p. 102.

59 In 1985, 86 out of 209 Labour MPs voted (41 per cent). In 1986, 108 Labour MPs voted (52 per cent).

4 The impact of the pro-research lobby

1 Leo Abse, 'The politics of in vitro fertilization in Britain', in S. Fishel and E. M. Symonds (eds.), *In Vitro Fertilization: Past, Present, Future* (Oxford: IRL Press, 1986), pp. 207–13, at p. 209; Steve Connor, 'MPs vote to ban embryo research', *New Scientist* 105 (21 February 1985), 3.

2 'Watchdog for embryo research', *New Scientist* 106 (4 April 1985), 5; Maxine Clarke, 'Voluntary authority set up', *Nature* 314 (4 April 1985), 397. For a detailed account of the establishment of the VLA, see Jennifer Gunning and Veronica English, *Human In Vitro Fertilization: A Case Study in the Regulation of Medical Innovation* (Aldershot: Dartmouth, 1993), chapters 3–4.

3 *IVF Research in the UK: A Report on Research Licensed by the Interim Licensing*

Authority (ILA) for Human In Vitro Fertilization and Embryology 1985–1989 (London: ILA, 1989), p. 1; see also Peter Thurnham, Commons, 23 April 1990, col. 58. For full bibliographical details of quotations from Hansard, see note 14 of the Introduction.

4 Progress: Campaign for Research into Reproduction, 'Constitution' (1985). In due course, Progress dropped the subtitle. In the main text, I have used only the shorter title. See also Mike Rayner, 'Experiments on embryos: stick to the facts', *New Scientist* 109 (27 February 1986), 54–5.

5 Progress: Campaign for Research into Reproduction, Minutes of the First Annual General Meeting, 16 June 1986, House of Commons, London.

6 See chapter 2, above.

7 Speakers in the ten major parliamentary debates (see note 14 of the Introduction) were classified as 'supporters of embryo research', as 'opponents of embryo research' or as 'undecided' at each stage in the sequence of debates by reference to their parliamentary testimony and their votes on the various Bills dealing with such research. The factors cited by each speaker as relevant to the evaluation of embryo research were noted and their frequency in each parliamentary session was recorded.

8 Department of Health and Social Security, *Human Fertilization and Embryology: A Framework for Legislation* (London: HMSO, 1987), Cm 259.

9 Lady Saltoun, Lords, 31 October 1984, col. 563.

10 In the opening debate in the Lords, all but one of the eighteen speakers opposed to embryo research argued explicitly, with Lady Saltoun, that the early human embryo has the same essential moral status as more biologically mature human organisms. In the opening debate in the Commons, twelve out of the nineteen opponents of embryo research emphasized the same point. In other speeches of opposition in the first Commons debate this point was present, but implicit. This remained a central criticism of embryo research throughout the remaining debates.

11 This theme was addressed by fourteen of the nineteen critics of embryo research in the first debate in the Commons and by eleven of the eighteen opponents of embryo research in the Lords.

12 Saltoun, Lords, 15 January 1988, cols. 1483–4.

13 See chapter 2 above for a discussion of the 'pre-embryo'; see also Michael Mulkay, 'The triumph of the pre-embryo: interpretations of the human embryo in parliamentary debate over embryo research', *Social Studies of Science* 24 (1994) 611–39. See also Anne McLaren, 'Why study early human development?', *New Scientist* 110 (24 April 1986), 49–52. The argument used to justify the use of the term 'pre- embryo' was that the fertilized human egg does not become a biologically organized individual until the formation of the first recognizable structural feature, that is, the 'primitive streak', which appears around day fourteen. Before that, the developing entity has no specialized cells, no differentiated tissues, no organs, no nervous system, and is still capable of dividing into two separate individuals. When the primitive streak appears, the cells that are to form the fetus separate from those that are to form the placenta and the

umbilical cord. These are the kinds of points that scientists would have made to Lady Saltoun and to other lay visitors on their visits to embryo research laboratories in order to convince them that the early human embryo is not an individual human being. The visitors would also have been told of the potential benefits of such research.

14 Saltoun, Lords, 31 October 1984, col. 560; see also Ann Winterton, Commons, 23 November 1984, col. 576.

15 Saltoun, Lords, 8 March 1989, col. 1574.

16 Ibid., cols. 1574–5.

17 The longest and most important debate in the Lords was that on 7 December 1989. In the Commons, the crucial debate was on 23 April 1990.

18 Jo Richardson, Commons, 23 April 1990, cols. 42–4.

19 See chapter 2 above; see also Andy Coghlan, 'Peers set the tone for Commons debate on embryo research', *New Scientist* 125 (17 February 1990), 19.

20 In the Commons in 1984, all seven speakers in favour of embryo research referred to the alleviation of infertility, whereas only three referred to control of genetic disease. In the Lords in 1984, the four supporters of embryo research all referred to the alleviation of infertility, but only two referred to control of genetic disease. This pattern was reversed during the closing stages of parliamentary debate. In the final Commons debate, twice as many supporters of embryo research referred to control over genetic disease as referred to the alleviation of infertility. In the Lords on 7 December 1989, twenty-one of the twenty-eight supporters of embryo research referred to control over genetic disease compared to fourteen who mentioned the alleviation of infertility.

21 Lord Caldecote, Lords, 7 December 1989, cols. 1056–7.

22 Only two paragraphs of the Warnock Report were devoted to the prevention of genetic defects, namely, paragraphs 12.15 and 12.16.

23 Viscount Buckmaster, Lords, 31 October 1984, col. 580.

24 See, for example, the contributions of the pro-researchers to the debate on the Unborn Children (Protection) Bill, 15 February 1985.

25 DHSS, *Human Fertilization*, note 8, paragraph 37; see also chapter 2 above.

26 See 'An appeal to embryologists', *Nature* 314 (7 March 1985), 11.

27 See McLaren, 'Why study?', note 13.

28 Thurnham, Commons, 23 April 1990, cols. 61–4.

29 Anne McLaren, 'Can we diagnose genetic disease in pre-embryos?', *New Scientist* 116 (10 December 1987), 42–7, at 47.

30 Edwina Currie, Commons, 23 April 1990, cols. 78–9.

31 Lord Jellicoe, Lords, 15 January 1988, col. 1466.

32 For full details of the Government legislation and the restrictions placed upon embryo research, see Derek Morgan and Robert G. Lee, *Human Fertilization and Embryology Act 1990: Abortion and Embryo Research, the New Law* (London: Blackstone, 1991); see also Gunning and English, *Human In Vitro Fertilization*, note 2, pp. 99–108.

33 Lord Kennet, Lords, 7 December 1989, cols. 1026–8.

5 Embryos in the news

1 Lord Ennals, Lords, 7 December 1989, col. 1015; Jo Richardson, Commons, 23 April 1990, col. 46. For full bibliographical details of quotations from Hansard, see note 14 of the Introduction.

2 A. E. P. Duffy, Commons, 23 April 1990, col. 55.

3 The following examination of newspaper coverage of embryo research during the concluding phase of parliamentary debate is based on a collection of press cuttings taken from newspapers throughout the period in which the Government Bill was passing through Parliament. These cuttings were obtained by Lincoln Hannah Ltd Mediascan for Dr Alan Handyside of the Hammersmith Hospital who kindly made them available for my use. Every relevant item was extracted from all national newspapers and leading provincial papers in Britain from the end of November 1989 to the beginning of July 1990. The total number of items was 218. Of these, 133 were routine items from staff reporters describing discussion of the Bill in Parliament. In addition, there were 85 more substantial items in the form of editorials, features or other kinds of presentation, often written by outside contributors, in which there was extended comment on and appraisal of embryo research and/or the technologies of assisted reproduction. These texts were very different in tone and content from the restrained and largely factual parliamentary reports. The five-to-two imbalance in favour of embryo research discussed in the main text was present only in this sub-set of 85 commentaries, editorials and special features. The routine reports on parliamentary debate displayed no particular bias either for or against embryo research. See Michael Mulkay, 'Embryos in the news', *Public Understanding of Science* 3 (1994), 33–51. For a general discussion of press coverage of science and technology, see Dorothy Nelkin, *Selling Science: How the Press Covers Science and Technology* (New York: W. H. Freeman, 1987). There is a brief account of the press reaction to 'test-tube babies' on pp. 50–1. See also Jose Van Dyck, *Manufacturing Babies and Public Consent: Debating the New Reproductive Technologies* (Basingstoke: Macmillan, 1995), pp. 62–6.

4 Sarah Franklin, 'Deconstructing "desperateness": the social construction of infertility in popular representations of new reproductive technologies', in M. McNeil, I. Varcoe and S. Yearley (eds.), *The New Reproductive Technologies* (Basingstoke and London: Macmillan, 1990), pp. 200–29. For documentation of clear parallels between Britain and Australia in the treatment by the press of assisted reproduction, see C. Noble and P. Bell, 'Reproducing women's nature: media construction of IVF and related issues', *Australian Journal of Social Issues* 27 (1992), 17–30.

5 *Daily Mail*, 19 April 1990. For a discussion of Robert Edwards's relationship with the *Daily Mail*, see Robert Edwards, *Life before Birth: Reflections on the Embryo Debate* (London: Hutchinson, 1989), pp. 12–15.

6 *The Independent*, 23 April 1990.

7 *Daily Mail*, 23 April 1990.

8 Maureen McNeil, 'Reproductive technologies: a new terrain for the sociology of technology', in McNeil, Varcoe and Yearley (eds.), *The New Reproductive Technologies*, note 4, pp. 1–26.

9 Edward Yoxen, 'Conflicting concerns: the political context of recent embryo research policy in Britain', in McNeil, Varcoe and Yearley (eds.), *The New Reproductive Technologies*, note 4, pp. 173–99.

10 'Action now', *Progress Bulletin No. 1* (September 1987).

11 See chapter 2 above.

12 *Statistical Analysis of the United Kingdom IVF and GIFT Data 1985–1990* (London: HFEA, 1992); *Third Annual Report* (London: HFEA, 1994), pp. 38–42. See also Lynda Birke, Susan Himmelweit and Gail Vines, *Tomorrow's Child: Reproductive Technologies in the 90s* (London: Virago, 1990), pp. 122–4, 127–8 and 135.

13 Michelle Stanworth (ed.), *Reproductive Technologies: Gender, Motherhood and Medicine* (Oxford: Polity Press, 1987); Patricia Spallone and Deborah Lynn Steinberg (eds.), *Made to Order: The Myth of Reproductive and Genetic Progress* (Oxford: Pergamon Press, 1987); Renate Klein, *The Exploitation of Desire: Women's Experiences with In Vitro Fertilization* (Victoria, Australia: Deakin University Press, 1989); Van Dyck, *Manufacturing Babies*, note 3, chapter 5.

14 This statement refers to the 218 cuttings on which my analysis is based. See note 3 above.

15 *Daily Mirror*, 19 April 1990. There is one clear story of failure in the **BABY SPECIAL**. But this story is headed 'How a husband suffers too' and is used, not to raise questions about assisted reproduction or embryo research, but to show that the pain of childlessness is not always confined to women. Van Dyck provides an example of an article emphasizing the high failure rate of IVF and drawing attention to the consequences for the women involved. This article was published in 1989 in the magazine *Ms*. Van Dyck stresses that this article was highly exceptional. See Van Dyck, *Manufacturing Babies*, note 3, p. 126.

16 Lene Koch, 'IVF – an irrational choice?', *Issues in Reproductive and Genetic Engineering* 3 (1990), 235–42.

17 *Sunday Times*, 10 December 1989. This article was probably intended to convince its readers that the Human Fertilization and Embryology Bill should be extended to cover the use of GIFT. This technique entails the extraction of eggs and the combination of sperm and eggs outside the womb. GIFT differs from IVF in that the mixture of sperm and eggs is transferred to the womb without waiting for fertilization to take place.

18 Ibid. See also Jennifer Gunning and Veronica English, *Human In Vitro Fertilization: A Case Study in the Regulation of Medical Innovation* (Aldershot: Dartmouth, 1993), p. 66.

19 Donald Gould, 'Steptonogo', *New Scientist* 79 (17 August 1978), 490.

20 *IVF Research in the UK: A Report on Research Licensed by the Interim Licensing Authority (ILA) for Human In Vitro Fertilization and Embryology 1985–1989* (London: ILA, 1989), p. 8.

21 This general line of argument was sometimes used by critics of embryo research in Parliament. See, for example, Ann Winterton, Commons, 4 February 1988. Some feminist critics also argued that research on the causes of infertility was preferable to research that produced intrusive and inefficient techniques designed to rectify infertility after women's reproductive capacity had been damaged by other factors. See Patricia Spallone, *Beyond Conception: The New Politics of Reproduction* (Basingstoke: Macmillan, 1989), chapter 3; Birke, Himmelweit and Vines, *Tomorrow's Child*, note 12, pp. 50–1.

22 This point is demonstrated clearly in Van Dyck, *Manufacturing Babies*, note 3, chapter 5, and especially pp. 125–6. Van Dyck also provides evidence of the selective use of the 'baby without blemish' story by the press and by the medical community of IVF practitioners.

23 Koch, 'IVF – an irrational choice?', note 16.

24 *Daily Telegraph*, 26 April 1990. Although the decisive vote had been taken by this date, the committee stage and the report stage of the Government Bill were still to come. See Gail Vines, 'Embryo Bill faces rocky ride in Commons', *New Scientist* 126 (26 May 1990), 18. The struggle between the opposing lobbies continued after the passage of the Bill and, indeed, continues still with reference to the membership and activities of the Human Fertilization and Embryology Authority: see chapter 9 below.

25 Out of eighty-five commentaries, only three or four gave voice to this kind of comprehensive denunciation of embryo research. For example, the *Sunday Telegraph*, 11 February 1990; the *Guardian*, 13 April 1990; *The Independent*, 23 April 1990.

26 *Daily Mail*, 16 July 1990. This item completed a story begun on 19 April 1990.

27 *Today*, 23 April 1990.

28 For a discussion of the difficulties involved in interpreting public opinion in relation to embryo research, see Geoffrey Hawthorn, 'The sociology of "public morality"', in *The CIBA Foundation, Human Embryo Research: Yes or No?* (London: Tavistock Publications, 1986), pp. 152–63.

29 *Evening Standard*, 9 February 1990.

30 *Evening Standard*, 19 April 1990.

6 Women and men

1 *Sunday Correspondent*, 11 February 1990. Unlike the situation in the Commons, it is impossible to be precise about the sexual imbalance in the House of Lords. This is because only a small proportion of its nominal membership of more than a thousand individuals actually participates in parliamentary debate. Nevertheless, it is clear that men always greatly outnumber women. See note 6 below.

2 Jo Richardson, Commons, 15 February 1985, col. 641. For full bibliographical details of quotations from Hansard, see note 14 of the Introduction.

3 Clare Short, Commons, 15 February 1985, col. 651.

4 The very phrase 'embryo research' tends to hide the fact that the female bearers of embryos are often centrally involved in the research. See the subsequent discussion in the main text. See also Gena Corea, *The Mother Machine: Reproductive Technologies from Artificial Insemination to Artificial Wombs* (London: The Women's Press, 1985).

5 These two major debates have been selected for particularly close inspection in order to facilitate precise comparisons between the speeches of men and women. These were the longest debates to occur during the period when the Government Bill was passing through Parliament. For a general discussion of the differences between women's and men's discourse, see Dorothy E. Smith, *The Everyday World as Problematic: A Feminist Sociology* (Milton Keynes: Open University Press, 1987), chapter 1. For a discussion of discursive differences in relation to reproduction, see Emily Martin, *The Woman in the Body: A Cultural Analysis of Reproduction* (Milton Keynes: Open University Press, 1987).

6 In the five major debates on embryo research in the Lords between 1984 and 1990, there were 120 speeches by men and 25 by women. In the five major debates in the Commons, there were 124 speeches by men and 29 by women. Although women spoke less often than men, they spoke significantly more frequently than would be expected on the basis of their numerical representation in the two Houses. In other words, it seems that choice of speakers was biased in favour of women in partial compensation for their low level of representation in Parliament; and perhaps also in implicit recognition of the claim that women had something especially important to say on this topic.

7 Kenneth Clarke, Commons, 23 April 1990, col. 31.

8 Ibid., col. 39.

9 *IVF Research in the UK* (London: ILA, 1989), p. 6.

10 Robert Edwards and Patrick Steptoe, *A Matter of Life: The Story of a Medical Breakthrough* (London: Hutchinson, 1980).

11 Lord Mackay, Lords, 7 December 1989, col. 1005.

12 Lord Ennals, Lords, 7 December 1989, col. 1013.

13 Michael Alison, Commons, 23 April 1990, col. 66.

14 Sir Bernard Braine, Commons, 23 April 1990, col. 47.

15 For detailed discussion of this issue, see Corea, *The Mother Machine*, note 4; and Patricia Spallone, *Beyond Conception: The New Politics of Reproduction* (Basingstoke: Macmillan, 1989).

16 Braine, Commons, 23 April 1990, col. 52.

17 Alan Amos, Commons, 23 April 1990, col. 106.

18 Ibid., col. 104.

19 Ibid., col. 107.

20 Whereas the Commons voted on embryo research in 1985 and 1986, the first vote on this topic in the Lords did not occur until 8 February 1990.

21 See Ann Widdicombe, Commons, 2 April 1990, col. 949; Dame Jill Knight, Commons, 2 April 1990, col. 958; Ann Winterton, 2 April 1990, col. 970.

22 Richardson, Commons, 23 April 1990, col. 44.

23 Audrey Wise, Commons, 23 April 1990, col. 92.

24 See Knight, Commons, 2 April 1990, col. 955.

25 Rosie Barnes, Commons, 23 April 1990, cols. 82–3.

26 Ibid., col. 83.

27 See Baroness Lockwood, Lords, 7 December 1989, col. 1033; Baroness White, Lords, 7 December 1989, col. 1045. See Smith, *The Everyday World*, note 5, p. 20.

28 Maria Fyfe, Commons, 23 April 1990, col. 64. See Martin, *The Woman in the Body*, note 5, chapter 8.

29 Harriet Harman, Commons, 23 April 1990, col. 119.

30 Barnes, Commons, 23 April 1990, col. 80. The speaker is referring here to the fact that some of the cells of the early embryo will eventually form the placenta. I interpret her remarks as a scornful comment on men's lack of familiarity with the messy details of human reproduction.

31 Baroness Llewelyn-Davies, Lords, 7 December 1989, cols. 1023–4.

32 Baroness Elles, Lords, 8 February 1990, cols. 973–4. Some women were offered free private-sector sterilization in exchange for their eggs during the late 1980s. When news of this practice became public, it was banned by the VLA. See Patricia Spallone, *Generation Games: Genetic Engineering and the Future for Our Lives* (London: The Women's Press, 1992), p. 214.

33 Elles, Lords, 8 February 1990, col. 974.

34 Lords, 8 February 1990, col. 976.

35 Lord Jenkin, Lords, 8 February 1990, cols. 976–7.

36 This may also explain the failure of the anti-research lobby to draw attention in the media to women's negative experiences with assisted reproduction. See chapter 5 above. Similarly, the anti-abortion lobby would have had little sympathy with the radical feminist critique of embryo research and assisted reproduction. It seems likely that feminist ideas concerning women's right to control their own bodies did influence parliamentary debate through the female members of the Labour Party. See chapter 3 above. There was, however, only one explicit reference to critical feminist analysis of embryo research in these debates. This was by the Labour MP Dale Campbell-Savours, Commons, 2 April 1990, cols. 969–70. Mr Campbell-Savours drew attention to the arguments against such research presented by the FINNRAGE group. The views of the feminist critics of embryo research were not mentioned by any of the female contributors to parliamentary debate. This may have been partly because these feminist critics were anti-research, yet also pro-abortion. Their views, therefore, would have been acceptable neither to the female supporters of embryo research in Parliament nor to its anti-abortionist opponents. The FINNRAGE group was said by Mr Campbell-Savours to be linked to the European socialist movement. This political affiliation would also have made these views seem alien to the Conservative female opponents of embryo research. See Corea, *The Mother Machine*, note 4; Spallone, *Beyond Conception*, note 15; Jose Van Dyck, *Manufacturing Babies and Public Consent:*

Debating the New Reproductive Technologies (Basingstoke: Macmillan, 1995), chapter 4.
37 Baroness Nicol, Lords, 7 December 1989, col. 1063.
38 Baroness Platt, Lords, 7 December 1989, cols. 1090 and 1092.

7 Science and religion

1 *Personal Origins: The Report of the Working Party on Human Fertilization and Embryology of the Board of Social Responsibility* (London: CIO Publishing, 1985), p. 1.
2 A detailed discussion of the response of the Roman Catholic Church is to be found in K. Boyd, B. Callaghan and E. Shotter, *Life before Birth: A Search for Consensus on Abortion and the Treatment of Infertility* (London: SPCK, 1986); see also G. R. Dunstan, 'The ethical debate', in S. Fishel and E. M. Symonds (eds.), *In Vitro Fertilization: Past, Present, Future* (Oxford: IRL Press, 1986), pp. 171–85.
3 The Archbishop of York spoke at length on these matters in the House of Lords on 15 January 1988, 7 December 1989 and 8 February 1990. See also the Archbishop's contribution to *The Times* on 23 April 1990, the day of the decisive debate in the Commons, entitled 'When Genesis is in conflict'. The Archbishop of York was trained as a scientist and was a university demonstrator in pharmacology at Cambridge from 1950 to 1953: see 'Last word' (editorial), *Independent on Sunday*, 11 February 1990.
4 For other parliamentary references to Galileo, see Lord Henderson, Lords, 8 March 1989, col. 1578 and Lord Flowers, Lords, 7 December 1989, cols. 1060–61. For full bibliographical details of quotations from Hansard, see note 8 below. For an early reference to Robert Edwards as the Galileo of embryo research, see Robert Edwards and Patrick Steptoe, *A Matter of Life: The Story of a Medical Breakthrough* (London: Hutchinson, 1980), p. 114. For another extended reference to Galileo linked to condemnation of the opponents of embryo research for their reliance on faith rather than reason, see Leo Abse, 'The politics of in vitro fertilization in Britain', in Fishel and Symonds (eds.), *In Vitro Fertilization*, note 2, pp. 207–13. For a critique of this use of Galileo, on the grounds that the cultural position of science in the seventeenth century was fundamentally different from that in the twentieth century, see Patricia Spallone, *Beyond Conception: The New Politics of Reproduction* (Basingstoke: Macmillan, 1989), p. 106.
5 Baroness Warnock, Lords, 7 December 1989, col. 1036. For full bibliographical details of quotations from Hansard, see note 8 below.
6 Lord Hailsham, Lords, 8 February 1990, col. 968.
7 Gareth Williams, 'Research on embryos', *New Scientist* 125 (20 January 1990), 70–1.
8 This chapter is based on examination of the following debates in *Parliamentary Debates* (Hansard), House of Lords, Fifth Series: Human Fertilization:

Warnock Report, vol. 456, 31 October 1984, 524–93; Human Fertilization and Embryology, vol. 491, 15 January 1988, cols. 1450–1508; Unborn Children (Protection) Bill, vol. 504, 8 March 1989, cols. 1538–80; Human Fertilization and Embryology Bill, vol. 513, 7 December 1989, cols. 1002–114; Human Fertilization and Embryology Bill, vol. 515, 8 February 1990, cols. 950–90.

9 This does not imply that the membership of the House of Lords is representative of British society as a whole; nor even that all significant religious groups are represented there. Nevertheless, the Upper House is one setting in which there were recorded discussions of embryo research involving scientists, representatives of various major religions and people who were neither scientists nor experts in religion. For observations on the representativeness of parliamentary membership in relation to this topic, see Ronald Frankenberg, 'Comment', *Current Anthropology* 33 (1992), 304–5. For criticism of the lack of direct representation from the scientific community in the House of Commons, see the remarks by Teresa Gorman, Commons, Human Fertilization and Embryology Bill, vol. 171, 23 April 1990, col. 118. For full bibliographical details of quotations from Hansard on debates in the House of Commons, see note 14 of the Introduction.

10 David Edge, 'Issues in science and religion', *Technology and Society* (University of Bath) 5 (1969), 13–21.

11 Ten speakers complimented the Marquess on the cogency of his speech and also, in most cases, in Lord Meston's words, for expressing 'what many of your Lordships clearly felt': 31 October 1984, col. 580. For other explicit examples of this Christian argument in the opening debate, see Lord Coleraine (col. 546), the Bishop of Norwich (col. 551), Lord Rawlinson (cols. 555–6), the Earl of Halsbury (col. 559), the Marquess of Lothian (col. 560), Lord Robertson (col. 567), the Earl of Longford (col. 575) and Baroness Masham (col. 577).

12 The Marquess of Reading, 31 October 1984, cols. 536–7.

13 The Bishop of Norwich, 31 October 1984, col. 553.

14 The Marquess of Lothian, 31 October 1984, col. 560. For other assertions of moral consensus regarding the immorality of embryo research in this debate, see Lord Rawlinson (col. 556), Lord Robertson (col. 567), Lord Tranmire (col. 574) and Viscount Buckmaster (col. 580).

15 The Bishop of Norwich argued that the 'gut reaction' of ordinary people to moral issues was important because 'quite often ordinary people get it right' (col. 553).

16 Lord Skelmersdale, who summed up for the Government, claimed an even larger majority for embryo research: 'The tally is that four out of the 21 speakers have come down firmly against research in any form of the word, whereas the rest are prepared to accept it' (15 January 1988, col. 1504). The distribution of support for and against embryo research among those who spoke on any particular occasion is, of course, only an approximate reflection of the balance of parliamentary opinion.

17 See, for example, Lord Meston, 31 October 1984, cols. 580–1 and Lord Prys-Davies, 31 October 1984, col. 584.

18 Lord Henderson, 15 January 1988, col. 1495. Lord Henderson was involved in organizing the parliamentary lobby in favour of embryo research. He acted as one of the whips for this lobby when the votes were cast in the Lords in 1990. His Lordship was wrong when he said that the Duke of Norfolk was the first speaker in this debate to use the words 'I believe'. In fact, the Archbishop of York, whom Lord Henderson praised for supporting embryo research without arguing from belief and who spoke before the Duke, used the words 'I believe' four times in his (somewhat longer) contribution.

19 See the remarks of the Earl of Longford, 15 January 1988, col. 1472.

20 Baroness Warnock, 15 January 1988, cols. 1468–70.

21 Edge, 'Issues in science and religion', note 10.

22 For other examples of this contrast at work, see Lord Prys-Davies, 15 January 1988, col. 1501; Lord Meston, 8 March 1989, col. 1544; Baroness Warnock, 8 March 1989, col. 1557; Lord McGregor, 7 December 1989, cols. 1016–17; Lord Houghton, 7 December 1989, col. 1058; Baroness Faithfull, 7 December 1989, col. 1099; Lord Sherfield, 7 December 1989, cols. 1100–1; and Lord Meston, 7 December 1989, cols. 1101–2.

23 For an example in the media of the accusation of 'woolly-minded' religious thought in relation to embryo research, see Matthew Parris, 'Searching for the source of life', *The Times*, 9 February 1990.

24 For further examples, see Baroness Ryder, 7 December 1989, col. 1066; Lord Rawlinson, 8 February 1990, col. 953; and Lord Hailsham, 8 February 1990, col. 966.

25 The Earl of Longford, 8 March 1989, cols. 1553–4.

26 Michael Mulkay, 'The triumph of the pre-embryo: interpretations of the human embryo in parliamentary debate over embryo research', *Social Studies of Science* 24 (1994), 611–39. For discussion of how the principle of the sanctity of life can be interpreted in various different ways, see Richard Dworkin, *Life's Dominion* (London: HarperCollins, 1993).

27 This was made particularly clear in the statement in the Lords by Lord Jellicoe, the head of the MRC, in response to the Government's White Paper: 15 January 1988, cols. 1463–4.

28 If we accept hypothetically the claim that the position of one side in the debate was based on reason, it follows that the other side can also claim to have been reasonable with regard to those moral arguments where the two sides were in agreement.

29 The opponents of embryo research were not necessarily opposed to other areas of scientific inquiry. For a specific example, see the speech by the Bishop of Ripon welcoming the work of scientists in general, but rejecting research involving human embryos: 8 March 1989, cols. 1546–9.

30 This is a paraphrase of part of the passage from Lord Henderson's speech quoted earlier: 15 January 1988, col. 1495.

31 Lady Warnock was referring here to arguments that addressed the good consequences of embryo research. These consequences, however, could not be taken into consideration by those who believed the ill-treatment of human embryos to

be inherently evil. For the latter, the pursuit of good ends could not justify the use of evil means. For an example of this argument, see the Earl of Lauderdale, 15 January 1988, col. 1487.

32 For other speakers who adopted this dismissive tone, see note 22.

33 15 January 1988, col. 1470.

34 Lord Kennet, 15 January 1988, cols. 1497–8.

35 Mary Warnock, *A Question of Life: The Warnock Report on Human Fertilization and Embryology* (Oxford: Blackwell, 1985), p. 60.

36 Lord Henderson, 15 January 1988, cols. 1494–5.

37 Ibid., col. 1495.

38 For other examples of explicit reliance on scientific authority, see Viscount Caldecote, 8 March 1989, col. 1570; Lord McGregor, 7 December 1989, cols. 1016–17; Baroness Lockwood, 7 December 1989, col. 1034; Viscount Caldecote, 7 December 1989, col. 1056; Baroness Carnegy, 7 December 1989, col. 1062; Baroness Platt, 7 December 1989, col. 1090; the Archbishop of York, 8 February 1990, col. 957; and Lord Bridge, 8 February 1990, col. 979.

39 See, for example, Lord McGregor, 7 December 1989, cols. 1016–17.

40 This assumption is implicit in the stereotyped contrast between science and religion. See Edge, 'Issues in science and religion', note 10.

41 In 1989, there were seventeen Members of the House of Lords who were scientists, plus the head of the MRC. This assessment is based on my reading of the information contained in *Dod's Parliamentary Companion*. It does not include individuals with a background in engineering. This figure may be compared with the twenty-six seats in the Lords reserved for Anglican bishops and archbishops. Nine of these scientist-peers spoke in the five major debates on embryo research, contributing a total of sixteen speeches (including three by the head of the MRC). Apart from the Earl of Halsbury, who opposed embryo research in his early speeches on religious grounds, these scientists spoke consistently in favour of embryo research. All of those who participated in the debates, including the Earl of Halsbury, voted for the continuation of embryo research in February 1990. Lord Flowers was the only scientist to refer to Galileo (7 December 1989, cols. 1060–1). The importance of moral commitment by scientists, as well as the importance of rational consideration of the evidence, was stressed in speeches by Lord Adrian, 7 December 1989, col. 1030; Lord Zuckerman, 7 December 1989, col. 1041; Lord Flowers, 7 December 1989, cols. 1060–1; Lord Butterfield, 7 December 1989, cols. 1063–5; and in two important speeches by Lord Walton, 7 December 1989, cols. 1051–5 and 8 February 1990, cols. 957–61. Most scientists did not enter the formal debate until December 1989. By this time, the shift in parliamentary opinion in the Lords was clearly established, and it may have seemed that there was no longer any need to attack religious opposition to embryo research with the vigour that had been appropriate in January 1988. This may be one reason why the lords of science were less aggressive towards their opponents than the lay speakers who had entered the fray at an earlier, and more uncertain, stage.

42 Lord Zuckerman, 7 December 1989, col. 1041.

43 For use of scientific findings by religious opponents of embryo research, see Lord Rawlinson, 31 October 1984, col. 555; the Marquess of Lothian, 31 October 1984, col. 560; Lord Robertson, 31 October 1984, col. 567; the Earl of Lauderdale, 15 January 1988, col. 1486; the Bishop of Ripon, 8 March 1989, col. 1548; the Duke of Norfolk, 7 December 1989, col. 1031; Lord Harvington, 7 December 1989, col. 1070; Lord Robertson, 7 December 1989, cols. 1093–4; and the Duke of Norfolk, 8 February 1990, col. 951. Whereas parliamentarians in favour of embryo research tended to cite the findings of embryologists to the effect that significant changes occur in the human embryo with the formation of the primitive streak at about fourteen days, those opposed to such research tended to cite the findings of geneticists to the effect that the genetic endowment of each human embryo is established at fertilization. For an attempt to reconcile these findings in a way that permits research on the early embryo, see Baroness Warnock, 15 January 1988, col. 1470. The subtle distinctions employed here strongly suggest that the nature of the early embryo was far from being a 'simple matter of fact'. For example: 'We must distinguish between the genetic information certainly already complete in the embryo and the individual life . . . The link is a causal link but not a link of identity. It is the lot of philosophers always to be thought to draw distinctions where none exist', and so on.

44 For example, see Viscount Buckmaster, 15 January 1988, cols. 1492–3; the Bishop of Ripon, 8 March 1989, col. 1547; Lord Longford, 8 March 1989, col. 1554; Lord Campbell, 8 March 1989, col. 1560; and Lord Carter, 7 December 1989, col. 1083. For statements on this matter by speakers in favour of embryo research, see Baroness Warnock, 8 March 1989, col. 1567 and by the Archbishop of York, 7 December 1989, col. 1019.

45 The Jewish community was represented by the Chief Rabbi, Lord Jakobovits, who argued against the creation of embryos specifically for experimental purposes, but in support of laboratory observation of spare embryos: 7 December 1989, cols. 1072–5. Not all members of the Jewish community agreed with Lord Jakobovits on this issue. The Islamic community was not represented directly in these debates. However, Viscount Buckmaster (31 October 1984, col. 580; 15 January 1988, col. 1493) and, later, Lord Campbell (8 March 1989, col. 1560) chose to speak on its members' behalf in condemnation of embryo research.

46 I. G. Barbour, 'Religion, values and science education', in B. Musschenga and D. Gosling (eds.), *Science Education and Ethical Values* (Washington, DC: Georgetown University Press, 1985), pp. 10–19, at pp. 13–14.

47 Lord Longford, 8 March 1989, cols. 1553–4.

48 Viscount Caldecote, 8 March 1989, cols. 1569–71.

49 For Catholic speakers in the crucial debate on 7 December 1989, see the Duke of Norfolk, col. 1031; Lord Longford, col. 1050; the Earl of Perth, col. 1085; Lord Robertson, cols. 1093–4; and the Earl of Cork and Orrery, col. 1095. For the position of the Catholic authorities, see Boyd, Callaghan and Shotter, *Life before Birth*, note 2. The existence of disagreement among Catholics in relation to embryo research is emphasized in Liam O'Brien, 'Status of embryos', *New Scientist* 124 (9 December 1989), 66.

50 Lord Carter, 7 December 1989, cols. 1082–3. See also Baroness Carnegy, 7 December 1989, col. 1062.

51 The report identifies two basic philosophical perspectives or patterns of interpretation in relation to the emergence of human personhood. The first is said to begin with existing persons and to proceed by tracing their development back to an initial point of origin such as the fertilization of the ovum by the sperm. The second approach is said to begin with consideration of the fertilized ovum and to proceed by searching for the attainment of attributes of personhood as the developing creature crosses certain biological thresholds, such as quickening, sentience or the appearance of the primitive streak. See *Personal Origins*, note 1, pp. 28–34. The Archbishop of York used this distinction in his defence of embryo research in the Lords on 15 January 1988, cols. 1460–3.

52 *Personal Origins*, note 1, p. 48.

53 The Bishop of Ripon, 8 March 1989, cols. 1546–7.

54 The Archbishop of York, 7 December 1989, col. 1019.

55 The Methodists, for example, tended to support embryo research. See Lord Soper, 31 October 1984, cols. 546–7; and Lord Walton, 7 December 1989, col. 1055.

56 Baroness Warnock, 7 December 1989, col. 1036.

57 See Lord Longford, 31 October 1984, col. 576; the Duke of Norfolk, 7 December 1989, col. 1032 and 8 February 1990, col. 951; and Lord Stallard, 8 February 1990, col. 970.

58 See Lord McGregor, 7 December 1989, col. 1017.

59 For details of scientific representation in the House of Lords, see note 41 above.

60 See Lord Jellicoe, 15 January 1988, col. 1467; Lord Rea, 15 January 1988, col. 1467; Lord Jellicoe, 8 March 1989, col. 1550; Lord Zuckerman, 7 December 1989, col. 1041; Lord Caldecote, 7 December 1989, col. 1056; Lord Flowers, 7 December 1989, col. 1061; and Lord Walton, 8 February 1990, cols. 959–60.

61 In the light of informal discussion with individuals involved in embryo research, I am inclined to think that scientists were less unified in private than in their public testimony.

62 The Archbishop of York was exceptional in giving firm and widely acknowledged guidance on this topic to Anglicans and others. However, he received little support from the rest of the Anglican leadership. See, for example, the comments by the Ven. George Austin, Archdeacon of York, in 'Cardinal reminder of moral absolutes' (letter), in the *Daily Telegraph*, 28 April 1990, concerning the failure of the Church of England to insist on moral absolutes in defence of the unborn child.

63 Lord McGregor, 7 December 1989, cols. 1017–19.

64 In addition to Lord McGregor, see Lord Ennals, 7 December 1989, col. 1013; Lord Hailsham, 7 December 1989, cols. 1022–3; Baroness Warnock, 7 December 1989, col. 1036; Lord Jellicoe, 7 December 1989, col. 1039; Baroness White, 7 December 1989, col. 1045; Baroness Carnegy, 7 December 1989, col. 1062; Lord Prior, 7 December 1989, col. 1088; and Lord Hailsham, 8 February 1990, cols. 966–8.

65 See, for example, Lord Soper, 31 October 1984, cols. 546–7; the Archbishop of York, 15 January 1988, cols. 1460–3; Lord Glenarthur, 7 December 1989, col. 1042; Lord Walton, 7 December 1989, col. 1051; Baroness Carnegy, 7 December 1989, col. 1062; and Lord Prior, 7 December 1989, col. 1088.

66 Warnock, *A Question of Life*, note 35, p. 60; Mulkay, 'The triumph of the pre-embryo', note 26; Christine Crowe, 'Whose mind over whose matter? Women, in vitro fertilization and the development of scientific knowledge', in M. McNeil, I. Varcoe and S. Yearley (eds.), *The New Reproductive Technologies* (Basingstoke and London: Macmillan, 1990), pp. 27–57.

67 See Lord Harvington, 8 February 1990, col. 963. See also the 'Discussion on ethical and judicial aspects of embryo research', *Human Reproduction* 4 (1989), 206–17, in which Jean-Paul Renard, of the Pasteur Institute, stated that he did not understand how the early diagnosis of human embryos would bring about the eradication of any genetic disease without the introduction of a total system of genetic control (213). If Renard is right, the attempt to control genetic disease through genetic screening of IVF embryos would require a massive extension in the use of IVF as well as a dramatic improvement in its success rate. These issues were hardly touched on in the course of parliamentary debate.

68 Baroness Warnock, 15 January 1988, col. 1469.

69 See, for example, Lord McGregor, 7 December 1989, col. 1017; Baroness Lockwood, 7 December 1989, col. 1034; Baroness Nicol, 7 December 1989, cols. 1062–3; Lord Shackleton, 7 December 1989, col. 1078; Baroness Platt, 7 December 1989, cols. 1090–2; the Archbishop of York, 8 February 1990, col. 957; and Lord Bridge, 8 February 1990, col. 979.

70 John Hedley Brooke, *Science and Religion: Some Historical Perspectives* (Cambridge: Cambridge University Press, 1991).

8 The myth of Frankenstein

1 Maureen McNeil, 'Reproductive technologies: a new terrain for the sociology of technology', in M. McNeil, I. Varcoe and S. Yearley (eds.), *The New Reproductive Technologies* (Basingstoke and London: Macmillan, 1990), pp. 1–26.

2 Aldous Huxley, *Brave New World* (London: Chatto & Windus, 1932). See also Jose Van Dyck, *Manufacturing Babies and Public Consent: Debating the New Reproductive Technologies* (Basingstoke: Macmillan, 1995). Van Dyck discusses in considerable detail the interpenetration of science, journalism and science fiction in relation to the new reproductive technology in the United States as well as in Britain.

3 Mary Shelley, *Frankenstein or The New Prometheus* (Oxford: Oxford University Press, 1969 [1818]). See also D. Glut, *The Frankenstein Legend* (Metuchen, New Jersey: Scarecrow, 1973); Langdon Winner, *Autonomous Technology: Technics-out-of-control as a Theme in Political Thought* (Cambridge: MIT Press, 1977); J. Smith (ed.), *Frankenstein: Case Studies in Contemporary Criticism* (Boston: St Martin's Press, 1992); J. Turney, 'In the grip of the monstrous myth', *Public Understanding of Science* 3 (1994), 225–31.

4 Andrew Tudor, 'Seeing the worst side of science', *Nature* 340 (24 August 1989), 589–92, at 589.

5 Andrew Tudor, *Monsters and Mad Scientists: A Cultural History of the Horror Movie* (Oxford: Blackwell, 1989).

6 C. P. Toumey, 'The moral character of mad scientists: a cultural critique of science', *Science, Technology and Human Values* 17 (1992), 411–37, at 434.

7 Department of Health and Social Security, *Human Fertilization and Embryology: A Framework for Legislation* (London: HMSO, 1987), Cm 259.

8 The *Sun*, 27 November 1987.

9 *Today*, 27 November 1987.

10 Dorothy Nelkin, *Selling Science: How the Press Covers Science and Technology* (New York: W. H. Freeman, 1987), p. 50.

11 'Shattered test tubes', *New Scientist* 116 (3 December 1987), 21.

12 *Nature* 330 (3 December 1987), 409.

13 Toumey, 'The moral character', note 6, 412.

14 Robert Edwards, *Life before Birth: Reflections on the Embryo Debate* (London: Hutchinson, 1989), pp. 69–70. The initial press reaction to the birth of Louise Brown in 1978 did involve considerable use of science fiction imagery. See Van Dyck, *Manufacturing Babies*, note 2, pp. 62–6.

15 This view of the disturbing influence of the Frankenstein myth seems to be widespread among scientists. See, for example, the suggestion by the eminent biologist Lewis Wolpert that one of the most useful things sociologists could do would be to explain why the 'Frankenstein image is so unrealistically persuasive in relation to genetic engineering': 'Response to Steve Fuller', *Social Studies of Science* 24 (1994), 745–7, at 745. Wolpert's proposal is another instance of a scientist using the supposed influence of science fiction to deny credibility to those who refuse to accept that scientific advance is necessarily beneficial.

16 Edwards, *Life before Birth*, note 14, p. 71.

17 For details of this material, see note 16 of the Introduction or note 3 of chapter 5.

18 *Independent on Sunday*, 29 April 1990.

19 See the discussion of press coverage of science and technology in Nelkin, *Selling Science*, note 10, and particularly pp. 50–1.

20 'Embryonic journey', *New Scientist* 124 (2 December 1989), 24.

21 The *Mirror*, 19 April 1990.

22 Baroness Masham, Lords, 31 October 1984, col. 576. For full bibliographical details of quotations from Hansard, see note 14 of the Introduction.

23 Ibid, col. 577.

24 Dale Campbell-Savours, Commons, 15 February 1985, col. 659.

25 The Earl of Lauderdale, Lords, 31 October 1984, col. 566.

26 The following speakers used science fiction imagery to criticize embryo research in the early debates: the Earl of Lauderdale, Lords, 31 October 1984, col. 566; Baroness Masham, Lords, 31 October 1984, col. 576; Norman St John-Stevas, Commons, 15 February 1985, col. 648; Dale Campbell-Savours, Commons, 15 February 1985, col. 659. The following speakers used science fiction imagery to

defend embryo research in the early debates: Michael Meacher, Commons, 23 November 1984, col. 534; Frank Dobson, Commons, 23 November 1984, col. 585; Jo Richardson, Commons, 15 February 1985, col. 643; David Crouch, Commons, 15 February 1985, col. 655; Michael Meacher, Commons, 15 February 1985, col. 686; Lord Rea, Lords, 15 January 1988, col. 1468. In the later debates, there were two passing references to science fiction by critics of embryo research: A. E. P. Duffy, Commons, 2 April 1990, col. 943; and William Benyon, Commons, 2 April 1990, col. 964. There were also two references to science fiction by supporters of embryo research in the Commons debate on 23 April 1990: Peter Thurnham, col. 64 and Edwina Currie, col. 77. In addition, in the debate in the Commons on 2 April 1990, Tam Dalyell, the political corre- spondent for *New Scientist*, asked the Minister to confirm that Mr Duffy's ref- erence to the eugenics of a brave new world was inappropriate in view of the fact that the legislation under consideration forbade any research that could lead in that direction (col. 977). The Minister for Health subsequently answered Mr Dalyell 'in the affirmative' (col. 982).

27 Dobson, Commons, 23 November 1984, col. 585.
28 Meacher, Commons, 23 November 1984, col. 534.
29 Meacher, Commons, 15 January 1988, col. 686.
30 Meacher, Commons, 23 November 1984, col. 536.
31 The logic underlying this technique for explaining away other people's beliefs is examined in detail in G. Nigel Gilbert and Michael Mulkay, *Opening Pandora's Box: A Sociological Analysis of Scientists' Discourse* (Cambridge: Cambridge University Press, 1984), chapter 4.
32 Pro-research rhetoric employed a twofold contrast between fact and fiction. On the one hand, it involved a comparison between two distinct genres or textual forms. On the other hand, it involved comparison between true and false asser- tions. These two contrasts often overlap, but they are not identical. See Michael Mulkay, *The Word and the World: Explorations in the Form of Sociological Analysis* (London: Allen & Unwin, 1985), pp. 10–12.
33 Sir Trevor Skeet, Commons, 4 February 1988, cols. 1225–7.
34 Bruce V. Lewenstein, 'Frankenstein or wizard: images of engineers in the media', *Engineering: Cornell Quarterly* 27 (1989), 40–8.
35 See, for example, Sir Gerard Vaughan, Commons, 23 November 1984, cols. 551–2; Jill Knight, Commons, 23 November 1984, cols. 565–6; William Cash, Commons, 23 November 1984, cols. 573–4; Sir Bernard Braine, Commons, 4 February 1988, cols. 1215–16; Kenneth Hind, Commons, 23 April 1990, col. 99; Alistair Burt, Commons, 23 April 1990, cols. 112–13; Lord Hanworth, Lords, 31 October 1984, cols. 545–6; Lord Rawlinson, Lords, 31 October 1984, cols. 555–6; the Earl of Perth, Lords, 7 December 1989, col. 1085; Lord Stallard, Lords, 8 February 1990, col. 970.
36 Tudor, 'Seeing the worst side', note 4, 591.
37 Toumey, 'The moral character', note 6; Michael Mulkay, 'Parliamentary ambivalence in relation to embryo research', *Social Studies of Science* 25 (1995), 149–63.

38 Tudor, *Monsters and Mad Scientists*, note 5.
39 Mary Warnock, *A Question of Life: The Warnock Report on Human Fertilization and Embryology* (Oxford: Blackwell, 1985). The Warnock Committee took the pragmatic view that it could only react to what it knew, and what it could realistically foresee (p. 5). There was clearly some debate about the length of the temporal perspective to be adopted. Warnock's subsequent account of the discussion of this topic suggests that some members of the committee tended to equate a long-term perspective with science fiction and that this term was used as a term of abuse. Lady Mary Warnock, 'Government commissions', in U. Bertazzoni, P. Fasella, A. Klepsch and P. Lange (eds.), *Human Embryos and Research: Proceedings of the European Bioethics Conference Mainz 1988* (Frankfurt/New York: Campus Verlag, 1990), pp. 159–68.
40 See Dr Charles Goodson-Wickes, Commons, 4 February 1988, col. 1237.
41 See, for example, Dafydd Wigley, Commons, 2 April 1990, cols. 945–8; Robert Key, Commons, 2 April 1990, cols. 952–4; Harriet Harman, Commons, 2 April 1990, cols. 978–81; Richardson, Commons, 23 April 1990, col. 47; Currie, Commons, 23 April 1990, cols. 77–9; Sir Ian Lloyd, Commons, 23 April 1990, cols. 94–8.
42 Meacher, Commons, 23 November 1984, col. 536.
43 Nelkin, *Selling Science*, note 10, p. 51.
44 Van Dyck, *Manufacturing Babies*, note 2, pp. 104–14 shows that embryo research and the new reproductive technology have been used in many different, and sometimes optimistic, ways in recent feminist fiction. The speakers in the British parliamentary debate, however, seem to have been unaware of this body of writing. Supporters of embryo research, of course, had no need to draw on the resources of utopian fiction because the research community provided them with a steady stream of authoritative science-based prophecies.

9 Embryo research and the slippery slope

1 This section reviews only the main factors involved in the victory of the pro-research lobby. It is not a comprehensive summary of the preceding chapters.
2 See chapters 5–7 in particular.
3 For further discussion of the rhetorics of hope and fear, see Michael Mulkay, 'Rhetorics of hope and fear in the great embryo debate', *Social Studies of Science* 23 (1993), 721–42; and Brian Bloomfield and Theo Vurdubakis, 'Disrupted boundaries: new reproductive technologies and the language of anxiety and expectation', *Social Studies of Science* 25 (1995), 533–51.
4 'Embryonic arguments', *New Scientist* 105 (14 February 1985), 2.
5 Human Fertilization and Embryology Authority, *Annual Report* (London: HFEA, 1992), p. 26.
6 Ibid.
7 For details of the Human Fertilization and Embryology Act and of the Human Fertilization and Embryology Authority, see Derek Morgan and Robert G. Lee,

Human Fertilization and Embryology Act 1990: Abortion and Embryo Research, the New Law (London: Blackstone, 1991), pp. 186–225.

8 The term 'pre-embryo' has dropped out of use since the passage of the 1990 Act. See the regretful comments of the chairman of the ILA in its last annual report: *The Sixth Report of the Interim Licensing Authority For Human In Vitro Fertilization and Embryology 1991* (London: ILA, 1991), p. 3. The idea that the human embryo undergoes a major transition around day fourteen was present in the Warnock Report and provided the justification for the fourteen-day limit on the experimental use of IVF embryos that was proposed in that document, and which was put into effect by the VLA shortly afterwards. The discussion of this topic in the Warnock Report, however, was brief and terminologically confused. The term 'pre-embryo' was introduced subsequently by the pro-research lobby to make the underlying idea clearer and more easily understood. See Michael Mulkay, 'The triumph of the pre-embryo: interpretations of the human embryo in parliamentary debate over embryo research', *Social Studies of Science* 24 (1994), 611–39.

9 Peter Garrett, 'Why we're afraid of the HFEA', *LIFE News*, No. 28 (Summer 1995), p. 8. This argument could have been applied equally well to the fourteen-day rule adopted by the VLA/ILA.

10 Rosalind Petchesky, 'Fetal images: the power of visual culture in the politics of reproduction', in M. Stanworth (ed.), *Reproductive Technologies: Gender, Motherhood and Medicine* (Cambridge: Polity Press, 1987), pp. 57–80.

11 'Cheating time', an edition of the BBC series *Horizon* broadcast on 13 January 1993. This view of early embryos destined for implantation must have been present in infertility clinics since the earliest days of IVF treatment. See the distinction between class 1 embryos and class 2 embryos in Michael Mulkay, 'Science and family in the great embryo debate', *Sociology* 28 (1994), 699–715.

12 'My twin darlings have made my life complete', *Woman's Own*, 26 August 1991, p. 14.

13 I have not carried out an extensive review of this literature. I should be surprised, however, if the existence of references to unborn children in infertility clinics was familiar to anti-abortionists, yet had not been mentioned in any of the sources I have consulted.

14 Early in 1995, the anti-abortion lobby in Parliament set up a new group, named Comment on Reproductive Ethics (CORE), to watch over the activities of the HFEA and the research and treatment it regulates. The main supporters of CORE are LIFE and the All-Party Parliamentary Pro-Life Group. See *Progress Bulletin*, No. 21 (Spring 1995), p. 2.

15 For a discussion of the notion of 'desperateness' in relation to assisted reproduction, see Sarah Franklin, 'Deconstructing "desperateness": the social construction of infertility in popular representations of new reproductive technologies', in M. McNeil, I. Varcoe and S. Yearley (eds.), *The New Reproductive Technologies* (Basingstoke and London: Macmillan, 1990), pp. 200–29.

16 See chapter 7 above.
17 Gail Vines, 'Pro-lifers attack fetal egg rules', *New Scientist* 143 (30 July 1994), 9.
18 *Sex Selection: Public Consultation Document* (London: HFEA, 1993), p. 7.
19 Ibid., pp. 8–9.
20 Ibid., p. 4.
21 Jose Van Dyck, *Manufacturing Babies and Public Consent: Debating the New Reproductive Technologies* (Basingstoke: Macmillan, 1995), p. 192. The HFEA arranges for groups of people from various backgrounds to meet to discuss topics of ethical concern to the Authority.
22 This quotation has been taken from *The Yorkshire Evening Press*, 21 March 1993. The BMA collectively rejected sex selection at its annual meeting in 1993: see Gail Vines, 'How far should we go?', *New Scientist* 141 (12 February 1994), 13.
23 Vines, 'How far?', note 22, 13.
24 HFEA, *Press Release 93–4*, 20 July 1993.
25 The source here is a letter from the chairman of the HFEA dated 15 July 1993 and addressed to the Parliamentary Under-secretary of State at the Department of Health. Copies of this letter were distributed with the HFEA's press release.
26 Ibid.
27 *Press Release 93–4*, note 24.
28 *Second Annual Report* (London: HFEA, 1993), p. 14.
29 Van Dyck, *Manufacturing Babies*, note 21, p. 187.
30 *Donated Ovarian Tissue in Embryo Research and Assisted Conception: Public Consultation Document* (London: HFEA, 1994), p. 2.
31 The document also contained proposals concerning the use of ovarian tissue, as distinct from eggs, from live donors. These proposals excited little public interest and have been omitted from the discussion in the main text.
32 *Public Consultation Document*, note 30, p. 2.
33 *Second Annual Report*, note 28, p. 14.
34 *Public Consultation Document*, note 30, p. 4.
35 Respondents were also asked to give their views on the procedures required for obtaining consent and on the need to increase the supply of eggs: ibid., p. 11.
36 Ibid., pp. 6–7.
37 Ibid., p. 10.
38 Dame Jill Knight, *Parliamentary Debates* (Hansard), House of Commons, Criminal Justice and Public Order Bill, vol. 241, 12 April 1994, cols. 158–9. See also the subsequent discussion, cols. 159–68; and House of Lords, Criminal Justice and Public Order Bill, vol. 555, 16 June 1994, cols. 1941–56.
39 Knight, Commons, 12 April 1994, cols. 158–9.
40 *Donated Ovarian Tissue in Embryo Research and Assisted Conception: Report* (London: HFEA, 1994), p. 9.
41 Vines, 'Pro-lifers attack', note 17, 9.
42 *Report*, note 40, p. 5.

43 Ibid.

44 Ibid.

45 Lord Walton, Lords, 16 June 1994, col. 1941.

46 *Report*, note 40, p. 2.

47 Ibid.

48 Ibid., p. 5.

49 Vines, 'Pro-lifers attack', note 17, 9.

50 Lord Walton, in his response to Dame Jill Knight's amendment, emphasized that the 'use of eggs from aborted fetuses may prove in the future, through research, to be useful in many other as yet unpredictable but widely acceptable ways': Lords, 16 June 1994, col. 1944. Jose Van Dyck maintains that it is fairly generally assumed by those engaged in research of this kind that people will get used to the idea of using fetal eggs for research and treatment, and that public opinion will gradually become more favourable. See Van Dyck, *Manufacturing Babies*, note 21, p. 188.

51 For analysis of this kind of reaction, see Bloomfield and Vurdubakis, 'Disrupted boundaries', note 3; and B. Bloomfield and T. Vurdubakis, 'Re-engineering the human: reproductive technologies and the spectre of Frankenstein', in D. Morgan and R. G. Lee (eds.), *Designer Babies?* (London: Gower, forthcoming).

52 In the eight major debates, this metaphor was used explicitly in 33 out of 189 speeches. It was accompanied by a cluster of supporting metaphors, such as 'the thin end of the wedge', 'the downward path', 'the foot in the door', 'crossing the Rubicon', 'looking over a precipice', and so on.

53 Baroness Warnock, Lords, 16 June 1994, col. 1471.

54 Kurt Kleiner, 'US to sanction embryo research', *New Scientist* 144 (8 October 1994), 5.

55 Andrew Kimbrell, *The Human Body Shop: The Engineering and Marketing of Life* (San Francisco and London: HarperCollins, 1993), pp. 124–5.

56 Ibid., p. 127.

57 Juliet Tizard, 'US considers embryo research legislation', *Progress Report*, No. 23 (Autumn 1995), 1. The Society of Assisted Reproduction Technology provides professional guidelines for its members. The American Medical Association intends to introduce new guidelines for researchers and clinicians in assisted reproduction by the end of 1995.

58 The high cost of IVF treatment means that it tends to be used disproportionately by higher-income groups.

59 Joseph Palca, 'Doing things with embryos', *Hastings Center Report*, January–February 1995, 5.

60 Kurt Kleiner, 'US finally faces up to embryo research', *New Scientist* 141 (12 February 1994), 8.

61 Palca, 'Doing things', note 59, 5.

62 'What research? Which embryos?, *Hastings Center Report*, January–February 1995, 36.

63 Ibid.

64 Kleiner, 'US to sanction', note 54, 5.
65 Daniel Callahan, 'The puzzle of profound respect', *Hastings Center Report*, January–February 1995, 39–40.
66 Ibid., 39.
67 Sheldon Krimsky and Ruth Hubbard, 'The business of research', *Hastings Center Report*, January–February 1995, 41–3, at 42.
68 This passage was written in November 1995.
69 'What research? Which embryos?', note 62, 36.
70 Andreas Frew, 'Congressional murder most foul', *New Scientist* 144 (29 October 1994), 67–8, at 68; and Palca, 'Doing things', note 59, 5. For a comprehensive examination of the pro-life movement in the USA, see Barbara Hinkson Craig and David M. O'Brien, *Abortion and American Politics* (Chatham, New Jersey: Chatham House Publishers, 1993).

Epilogue

The list of references below is an attempt to identify some of the public sources that seem to have influenced Mrs Everyman's dream. Fragments from several of these texts appear with only minor changes at various points in the dream sequence. The impact of other items has been less direct. But the dreamer's imagination has reworked all this material, changing its context and exploring its implications in a personal response to the complex mixture of beliefs and cultural practices that has grown up around IVF, embryo research and related activities.

J. H. Barnsley, *The Social Reality of Ethics* (London: Routledge & Kegan Paul, 1972).
U. Bertazzoni, P. Fasella, A. Klepsch and P. Lange, *Human Embryos and Research* (Frankfurt/New York: Campus Verlag, 1988).
R. G. Edwards et al., 'Discussion on ethical and judicial aspects of embryo research', *Human Reproduction* 4 (1989), 206–17.
R. G. Edwards and D. J. Sharpe, 'Social values and research in human embryology', *Nature* 231 (14 May 1971), 87–91.
G. Holton, *Thematic Origins of Scientific Thought* (London/Cambridge, Mass: Harvard University Press, 1988).
T. Iglesias, '*In vitro* fertilization: the major issues', *Journal of Medical Ethics* 1 (1984), 32–37.
A. McLaren, 'Why study early human development?', *New Scientist* 110 (24 April 1986), 49–52.
   'Can we diagnose genetic disease in pre-embryos?', *New Scientist* 116 (10 December 1987), 42–7.
M. Mulkay, *Sains dan Sosiologi ilmu Pengetahuan* (Kuala Lumpur: Dewan Bahasa dan Pustaka, 1990).

Index